Paying for Health Care after Age 65

Choices and Challenges:
An Older Adult Reference Series
Elizabeth Vierck, Series Editor

Housing Options and Services for Older Adults,
Ann E. Gillespie and Katrinka Smith Sloan

Mental Health Problems and Older Adults,
Gregory A. Hinrichsen

Paying for Health Care after Age 65,
Elizabeth Vierck

Forthcoming

Legal Issues and Older Adults,
Linda Josephson Millman and Sallie Birket Chafer

Older Workers, Sara E. Rix

Travel and Older Adults, Allison St. Claire

Volunteerism and Older Adults, Mary K. Kouri

Paying for
Health Care
after Age 65

Elizabeth Vierck

Choices and Challenges: An Older Adult Reference Series

ABC-CLIO

Santa Barbara, California
Oxford, England

Cover Design/Graphein

Library of Congress Cataloging-in-Publication Data

Vierck, Elizabeth, 1945–
    Paying for health care after age 65 / Elizabeth Vierck.
      p. cm.—(Choices and challenges)
    Includes bibliographical references and index.
    1. Medicare—Handbooks, manuals, etc. 2. Medigap—Handbooks,
  manuals, etc. I. Title. II. Series.
    HD7102.U4V54 1990   344.73'0226—dc20 [347.304226]   90-40320

ISBN 0-87436-095-1 (alk. paper)

97 96 95 94 93 92 91 90   10 9 8 7 6 5 4 3 2 1

ABC-CLIO, Inc.
130 Cremona Drive, P.O. Box 1911
Santa Barbara, California 93116-1911

Clio Press Ltd.
55 St. Thomas' Street
Oxford, OX1 1JG, England

This book is Smyth-sewn and printed on acid-free paper ∞.
Manufactured in the United States of America

In memory of my grandparents, Mayme and Earl Amadon.
To my sister and brother, Sally and Charles.
Again to Craig and Mom.

Contents

List of Tables and Figures, xiii
Acknowledgments, xv
Introduction, xvii
How To Use This Book, xxiii

PART ONE   **Paying for Health Care**

Chapter 1:   An Overview, 5

Medicare Facts, 5

Introduction, 5

History of the Medicare Program, 6

Medicare's Limitations, 8

Eligibility for Medicare, 9

Medicare's Disability Benefits, 10

Medicare Assistance Programs, 16

The Medicare Handbook, 17

Things to Remember, 18

Chapter 2:   Medicare Part A, 19

Medicare Part A Facts, 19

Introduction, 20

Inpatient Hospital Care, 20

Skilled-Nursing-Facility (SNF) Care, 26

Home Health Care, 29

Hospice Care, 33

Chapter 3:   **Medicare Part B, 35**

Medicare Part B Facts, 35

Introduction, 35

The Health Services Network, 36

Doctors' Services, 37

Chapter 4:   **Paying for Medicare Coverage
and Collecting Benefits, 43**

Medicare Costs and Reimbursement Facts, 43

Introduction, 44

Part B Costs, 44

Purchasing Medicare Coverage, 45

Enrolling in Part B When Eligible for Part A, 46

Using the Assignment Method for
Part B Services, 46

Collecting Payment from Medicare, 51

Notice of Payment by Medicare, 57

When a Relative Dies, 58

How Approved Charges Are Determined, 59

When Medicare Is the Secondary Payer, 62

Chapter 5:   **Beneficiaries' Rights To Appeal
Medicare Claims, 63**

Facts on Medicare Appeals, 63

Introduction, 63

Who Can Appeal, 65

Part A Appeals, 65

Part B Appeals, 75

Part A and Part B Appeals, 78

Chapter 6:   **Supplementing Medicare, 85**

Facts on Supplemental Insurance, 85

Introduction, 86

Covering Out-of-Pocket Health-Care Costs, 87

Continuing Group Health Insurance, 87

Coverage for Age 65-plus Workers, 88

Purchasing Supplemental Health Insurance, 88

Health Maintenance Organizations, 96

Preferred Provider Organizations, 103

Medicaid Benefits, 104

Financial Assistance for Low-Income Medicare Beneficiaries, 107

Veterans' Benefits, 107

Catastrophic or Major Medical Insurance, 109

Indemnity and Other Limited Policies, 109

Insurance Options Prior to Becoming a Medicare Recipient, 110

Chapter 7:   **Paying for Long-Term Care, 111**

Facts on Long-Term Care, 111

Introduction, 111

The Need for Long-Term Care, 112

Help in the Home, 113

Nursing Homes, 128

Other Residential Options for
Long-Term Care, 133

Long-Term-Care Insurance, 133

Chapter 8:   Saving Health-Care Dollars, 139

Facts on Saving Health-Care Dollars, 139

Introduction, 139

Checklist for Reducing Health-Care Costs, 140

Health-Promotion Techniques, 140

Medical-Expense Deductions for
Federal Taxes, 141

Federal Tax Credits for Dependent Care, 142

When a Relative Dies, 143

Second Surgical Opinions, 143

Ambulatory Emergency Centers, 143

Saving Money on Prescription Drugs, 144

Saving Money on Medical Care, 145

Clinics and Doctors To Stay Away From, 145

Sources for Part One, 147

PART TWO   Resources

Chapter 9:   Who's Who in Health Care, 153

General Medical Care, 153

Dental Care, 155

Eye Care, 156

Muscle, Bone, and Foot Care, 157

Mental-Health Care, 157

Other Medical Care, 158

Chapter 10: **Directory of Organizations, 161**

General Organizations, 161

Government Agencies, 171

Health, Social Service, and Long-Term-Care Organizations, 194

Health and Social Service Professional Organizations, 213

Self-Help Organizations, 217

State Health-Insurance Counseling Programs, 221

Chapter 11: **Reference Material, 227**

Books, 227

Pamphlets, 236

Articles, 239

Periodicals, 239

State Publications on Medicare, Supplemental Plans, and Long-Term-Care Insurance, 241

Nonprint Materials, 258

Glossary, 261
Index, 279

Tables and Figures

Table 1.1   Medicare Benefits and Costs, 17
Table 4.1   Saving Money through Assignment: A Comparison of Two Claims for the Same Procedure, 50
Table 4.2   Medicare Claims Processing, 57
Table 5.1   Major Diagnostic Categories Used in Medicare's Payment System, 70
Table 5.2   Top Ten Diagnostic Related Groups (DRGs) with the Most Discharges, 71
Table 6.1   Medicare-Approved HMOs by Region, 98
Table 6.2   A Comparison of Medicare and Medicaid, 104

Figure 1.1   Sample of a Medicare Card, 9
Figure 1.2   Applications To Purchase Medicare Coverage. Form HCFA-18 F5, 11
Figure 2.1   An Important Message from Medicare, 24
Figure 4.1   Application for Medical Insurance under Medicare. Form HCFA-40B, 47
Figure 4.2   Sample of a Medicare Benefit Notice, 51
Figure 4.3   Request for Medical Payment. Form HCFA-1490S, 53
Figure 4.4   Medicare Medical Insurance Claims Record. Form SSA-3596, 56
Figure 4.5   Sample Medicare Claims Information, 58
Figure 4.6   Sample Explanation of Medicare Benefits (EOMB), 59
Figure 4.7   Request for Information. Form HCFA-1660, 60
Figure 5.1   Request for Reconsideration for Part A Benefits. Form HCFA-2649, 67
Figure 5.2   Request for a Hearing: Part A Benefits. Form HA-5011, 68

Figure 5.3   Request for Social Security Appeals Council
              Review. Form HA-520, 69
Figure 5.4   Request for Review of Part B Medicare Claim.
              Form HCFA-1964, 77
Figure 5.5   Request for Medicare-Carrier Hearing. Form
              HCFA-1965, 79
Figure 5.6   Agreement To Have Representation at Hearing.
              Form SSA-1696, 80

Acknowledgments

No nonfiction book is ever written by the author alone. It is impossible to list in this small space the countless names of people I interviewed for this volume during the past year. Many experts on financing health care for the elderly freely gave their time and expertise to answer endless questions and to supply me with mountains of materials. I am indebted to them for their invaluable contributions. I would particularly like to thank my friend Susan Hellman, director of Colorado's Senior Health Insurance Counseling Project, for her help above and beyond the call of duty. In addition, Carla McDonald assisted me in compiling sections of Part Two, and I would like to thank my editor, Laurie Brock, for her enthusiastic support of the entire Choices and Challenges series. I would also like to thank Judyl Mudfoot, project editor at ABC-CLIO, for her brilliant design for the series. Lastly, I would like to thank my husband, Craig Boyle, who, as always, is my best champion.

This book is, in part, the result of a project funded through a Health Care Financing Administration Small Business Innovation Research grant (contract no. 500-88-0039) awarded to the author.

Introduction

In 1984 Mr. Devon's daughters, Rose and Caroline, became concerned that their father was developing Alzheimer's disease and would need nursing-home care. Their first thought, as they set out to plan for their father's care, was "Well, we don't have to worry about the cost, Medicare will cover it." Mr. Devon was admitted to a nursing home in 1986, and his daughters have been paying an average of $32,000 a year out of their own pockets for his care.

In order to keep health-care costs down, Mrs. Klein shops carefully for physicians and other health providers who accept Medicare's approved charge on their claims (commonly referred to as "accepting assignment"). However, when Mrs. Klein recently went into the hospital for surgery, several doctors whom she had never met, including an anesthesiologist and a pathologist, performed services for her. None of these doctors accepted assignment.

After her surgery Mrs. Klein received more than 50 documents called "explanation of benefits" from Medicare and her supplemental insurance carrier. It took her more than eight hours just to sort out the documents, and, in the end, she still had no idea what Medicare and her private insurance company had paid to the hospital, her doctor, and other providers, or how much she owed. However, one thing was clear: Mrs. Klein was stuck with paying the excess charges of anesthesiologist, the pathologist, and the other health providers who did not accept assignment.

Mrs. Dolores Smith was scrimping to pay premiums on eleven Medicare supplemental policies. When asked why she had purchased so many policies, she described one of the greatest fears of today's seniors: "I don't want to burden my kids if I have to go into a nursing home." Unfortunately, because of the insurance policies' confusing legal language, Mrs. Smith did not realize that *none* of the policies she had purchased covered the costs of long-term care in a nursing home.

Paying for Health Care after Age 65 addresses the concerns of older adults such as Mr. Devon, Mrs. Klein, Dolores Smith, and the relatives, friends, and professionals who care about them. Let's take a brief look at some of the complexities of the programs that these individuals must contend with once they reach the age of eligibility for Medicare.

When they reach their sixty-fifth birthday, Uncle Sam mails most older Americans a Medicare card, good for admission to America's health-care system for the remaining lifetime of the holder. That is the good news. The bad news is twofold: (1) because of Medicare's mazelike structure, very few card holders understand exactly what it purchases or how to use it effectively, and (2) the card is a bit of a mixed blessing—it has a great many restrictions, limitations, and hidden costs attached to it.

The Medicare Maze

Since its birth more than 25 years ago as part of Lyndon Baines Johnson's Great Society program, Medicare has evolved into one of the most complex government programs in the world. As such, it is also the cornerstone of health care for older adults. Many tongue-in-cheek attempts have been made to describe Medicare's complexity. Medicare has been referred to as the Two-Headed Monster (Medicare Part A and Part B), the Medicare Maze, Medibabble, and Mediboggle, to name a few. And many jokes have been made about Medicare's alphabet-soup approach to health care (PPS, DRGs, Part A, Part B, SNFs, NFs, EOMBs, and so on).

Unfortunately, Medicare's knotty complexity complicates beneficiaries' dependence on the program, specifically because the need for health care in later life is so substantial. One of the paradoxes of aging is that tremendous gains in life expectancy in this century have resulted in a postponement of many chronic health-care problems. For example:

> More than four out of five persons 65 and over have at least one chronic condition, and multiple conditions are commonplace in later life.
>
> On the average, older persons visit a physician eight times a year.
>
> Slightly more than a third of all older persons are hospitalized at least once in a year.
>
> Nearly half of persons over 65 have arthritis, about 40 percent have high blood pressure, and more than 25 percent have heart disease.

While the need for Medicare in later life is obvious, misconceptions about it and its related programs are far more common than an understanding of them. A survey by the American Association of Retired Persons (AARP) found that the majority of older adults did not know what services Medicare actually covered. Indeed, many people confuse Medicare and Medicaid, two programs that are as different as pudding and Jello.

Perhaps the most common misconception held by most Americans is that after age 65 "insurance pays" when illness strikes. According to a 1986 Gallup poll, three-quarters of Americans *overestimate* the proportion of health care that Medicare pays. In fact, Medicare paid for only 40 percent of the health expenses of older Americans in 1988. Other private sources, Medicaid, and other government sources covered only another 12 percent.

Much of the misunderstanding about Medicare is about as easy to clear up as eating alphabet soup with chop sticks. The program is just too complicated to explain easily. Medicare is a $100 billion program benefitting 30 million older adults and another 3 million disabled persons. It consists of two parts, A and B, and each part is governed by a tangle of rules and regulations that determine what Medicare will and will not cover. For example, the formulas that are used to determine what portion of medical expenses Medicare will pay are so complicated that the majority of beneficiaries do not even try to figure them out. This means that if there are problems or mistakes on a bill the Medicare recipient is generally not aware of them. In fact, the system is so complex that large numbers of beneficiaries do not seek reimbursement, adding up to $40 million in unre-imbursed doctor's bills annually. This is known among health-policy analysts as the "shoebox effect," in which beneficiaries pay the doctors' bills themselves and stuff the reimbursement forms in shoeboxes, rather than having to grapple with filling them out and sending them in. The "shoebox effect" is but one result of a precarious and mazelike system that generally leaves the beneficiary in the dark.

Medicare's Restrictions, Limitations, and Costs

Unfortunately, Medicare is also not meeting the health-care needs of older adults as its architects had originally designed it to do. Medicare, by definition, has many restrictions and limita-tions. As mentioned earlier, it covers less than half of the total costs of health care for older adults. Most significantly, Medicare does not cover the costs of the major catastrophic expense of the elderly—long-term care. Surveys have shown that this fact is frequently misunderstood by older Americans—most individu-als assume that Medicare will at least cover the cost of long-term care in a nursing home.

Almost 25 years after the founding of Medicare, significant costs remain for the older consumer:

> The average older American is spending about 15 percent of his or her income on health care. (Fifteen percent is the level most economists and policy analysts use to define when health costs become catastrophic.)

> Out-of-pocket costs for Medicare beneficiaries are proportionately *higher* than they were before Medicare was enacted in 1965.

> The monthly Medicare Part B premium has risen in three years from $17.90 in 1987 to $28.60 in 1990. And this increased cost is occurring without any added coverage benefits that were added by the Medicare Catastrophic Coverage Act were repealed in 1989.

Certainly this is a failure in our country's health policy. Older health-care consumers have no choice but to come up with the necessary dollars to cover burgeoning health costs.

Adding to the Medicare quagmire is the fact that the programs that supplement or complement it are often as baffling as Medicare itself. Because of Medicare's limitations, these programs, such as Medicaid and medigap insurance, are necessary protections against astronomical health-care costs. However, every state takes a different approach to regulating them. In Massachusetts, for example, older residents have three basic medigap policies to choose from, while older Coloradans must select from more than 90 policies. And Medicaid, the health-insurance program for those with low incomes, also varies tremendously by state. In fact, an individual living in one state and receiving comprehensive medical care and home health care services might not even qualify for another state's Medicaid program.

Paying for Health Care after Age 65

Paying for Health Care after Age 65 is a simplified guide to these issues. As a reference book, it provides a boiled-down explanation of Medicare, its related programs, and other issues relevant to the costs of health care after age 65.

Paying for Health Care after Age 65 provides much more information than Medicare or any other government source makes available for beneficiaries: how and when to appeal a Medicare claim, for example, or which long-term-care services Medicare, Medicaid, and other government sources are most likely to cover and when. *Paying for Health Care after Age 65* also explains what to look for in Medicare supplements, what long-term-care services are available in communities across the country, and how to choose a long-term-care policy. It also provides a potpourri of important information about saving health-care dollars, such as federal tax credits for dependent care or when a relative is responsible for the medical bills of a deceased family member. This book also includes an extensive resource section with a detailed annotated bibliography, a list of national and state organizations, a guide to types of health-care professionals, and a glossary. This section represents the first time that such extensive resources on the topic have been compiled and published under one cover.

One caveat must be mentioned. The Medicare program is in flux, and its benefits and costs could change within the next year or two. First, it is possible that some limited benefits such as respite care or regular mammograms that were included in the Medicare Catastrophic Coverage Act, which was repealed in 1989, will be put back into the program. Second, because Medicare is facing a deficit, sometime near the turn of the century beneficiary costs could be increased by Congress in order to collect revenues. Third, Congress could pass legislation to help older adults pay for their long-term care. Any one of these amendments would change the benefits that are described in the following pages, and these issues are worth following closely in the 1990s. In addition, Congress may also adopt physician payment reforms that will alter the way physicians are reimbursed and consumer protection provisions for purchasers of Medicare supplemental insurance. If there are any questions regarding these possible changes, the reader may want to contact relevant organizations listed in Part Two of this book.

How To Use This Book

Each book in the Choices and Challenges series provides a convenient, easy-access reference tool on a specific topic of interest to older adults and those involved with them, including caregivers, spouses, adult children, and gerontology professionals. The books are designed for ease of use, with a generous typeface, ample use of headings and subheadings, and a detailed index.

Each book consists of two parts, which may be used together or independently:

A narrative section providing an informative and comprehensive overview of the topic, written for a lay audience. The narrative can be read straight through or consulted on an as-needed basis by using the headings and subheadings and/or the index.

An annotated resource section that includes a directory of relevant organizations; recommended books, pamphlets, and articles; and software and videos. Where appropriate, the resource section may include additional information relevant to the topic. This section can be used in conjunction with or separately from the narrative to locate sources of additional information, assistance, or support.

A glossary defines important terms and concepts, and the index provides additional access to the material. For easy reference, entries in the resource section are indexed by both topic and title or name.

PART
ONE

Paying for
Health Care

The first six chapters of this book are a comprehensive look at the Medicare program. Chapters 1 through 3 provide basic facts on Medicare and how it works; Medicare's hospital program, Part A; and its medical insurance, Part B. Chapter 4 covers paying for Medicare coverage and collecting payment from Medicare. Chapter 5 explains Medicare appeals, which are the legal means that Medicare beneficiaries or providers may use to question Medicare's reimbursement decisions.

The remaining chapters of Part One focus on filling in Medicare's gaps. Chapter 6 discusses purchasing supplemental health insurance, joining an HMO, becoming eligible for Medicaid benefits, and other options for supplementing Medicare. Chapter 7 looks at options for financing long-term care. And finally, Chapter 8 is a potpourri of consumer tips for saving health-care dollars.

Chapter 1

An Overview

- Medicare provides health coverage for 97 percent of Americans 65 and older.

- While Medicare is indispensable to older health consumers, it covers only about 40 percent of their health-care costs.

- Medicare does not cover the costs of long-term care in a nursing home or at home. Expenses for such care are the greatest threat to the economic security of the elderly.

- Medicare is a two-part program. Part A, hospital insurance, and Part B, medical insurance, work together to provide a single comprehensive insurance program.

- Congress has been in turmoil during the past few years, attempting to provide expanded benefits to Medicare beneficiaries. First, in 1988 Congress passed the Medicare Catastrophic Coverage Act, and then, in 1989 it repealed it.

Introduction

Enacted in 1965, Medicare is a $100-billion federal health-insurance program for persons 65 and older who are eligible for Social Security or Railroad Retirement. Medicare is run by the federal Health Care Financing Administration (HCFA), part of the U.S. Department of Health and Human Services. It provides hospital and medical coverage for 97 percent of the older population, equalling about 40 percent of total health-care costs for older adults. In 1989, 29.4 million people age 65 or older were enrolled in Medicare Part A. Of those, it is estimated that 6.7 million aged received reimbursed services. There are 29.2 million aged also enrolled in Part B, and 23.6 million received reimbursed services. In addition, 3.2 million disabled are enrolled in Part A, and 2.9 million are enrolled in Part B.

Medicare coverage yields significant savings for beneficiaries. In 1987 the average amount of reimbursement per Medicare beneficiary served was $2,870. Medicare's funding is provided by three sources. Medicare Part A's Hospital Insurance Trust Fund is financed through a payroll tax, and Part B is financed through beneficiary premiums and general revenues. Unhappily, the Hospital Insurance Trust Fund is expected to run dry in the early part of the next century, which will create a major policy issue for Congress.

Medicare's architects designed an indirect program of finance and delivery as opposed to a direct program such as the U.S. military service, which directly oversees its health services. Medicare beneficiaries are responsible for locating services. And the HCFA does not directly reimburse patients or providers, but pays them through a system of intermediaries and carriers.

History of the Medicare Program

The first glimpse of the Medicare program came into public view in 1935 when Congress considered passing national health insurance as part of the Social Security Act. During this time congressional supporters of health insurance for all Americans were responding to the fact that health insurance was primarily sponsored by employers, so that all nonworkers, including the elderly, had little protection against catastrophic health-care costs. Nevertheless, fierce objections from the American Medical Association (AMA) and conservative members of Congress derailed passage of a public health-insurance program.

During the next couple of decades further unsuccessful attempts were made to pass similar bills, and finally, during the 1950s health insurance for the elderly became a hot topic on Capitol Hill. In 1958 a bill that was the forerunner of Medicare was introduced by Congressman Aime Forand of Rhode Island.

Ironically, during this time there was strong opposition by the AMA and others to include physician payments in Medicare. Today physician payments make up 28 percent of the Medicare budget.

In 1959 a newly established Senate Committee on Aging held hearings on the topic, bringing national attention to the issue. In response, many elderly and their families answered an appeal to "write their congressman," and Capitol Hill offices bulged with stacks of mail encouraging passage of health insurance for the elderly. Finally, Congress took a first step and in 1960 passed the Kerr-Mills Act, which provided medical assistance to the aged poor. However, the low-income limitations of the act left the issue largely unsettled.

When John F. Kennedy was inaugurated as president in 1961, he brought strong support of health insurance for all elderly with him to the White House, but he did not live to see it signed into law. He could not marshal enough votes for passage of the bill. Eventually, the time was ripe for change when the Democrats swept the Congress in 1964. And finally, on July 30, 1965, Medicare (Title XVIII of the Social Security Act) was signed into law by President Lyndon Baines Johnson.

There were three parts to the new health-insurance program that was developed by Congressman Wilbur Mills, chairman of the House Ways and Means Committee: (1) compulsory hospital insurance (Part A of Medicare), (2) voluntary insurance for physicians' bills (Part B of Medicare) and, (3) expanded assistance to the states for medical care for the poor (Medicaid). Passage of Title XVIII's Part A of Medicare marked the first time that Congress put its stamp of approval on a social health-insurance program as opposed to medical assistance for the poor.

During the past two and a half decades Medicare has covered a large share of health-care costs for millions of older and disabled Americans. Today it is the cornerstone of health care for persons over age 65.

Repeal of the Medicare Catastrophic Coverage Act

Congress has been in turmoil during the past few years, in its attempt to provide expanded benefits to Medicare beneficiaries. First, in 1988 Congress passed the Medicare Catastrophic Coverage Act, and then, in 1989 it repealed it. Fortunately, two important benefits for older persons with low incomes remain from the passage of the 1988 Medicare Catastrophic Coverage Act (MCCA). They are income and asset protection for a person who has a spouse in a nursing home and payment by Medicaid of premiums and deductibles for very low-income Medicare beneficiaries who are not presently covered by Medicaid.

The repeal of the MCCA demonstrated the tremendous political power of older adults. In truth, if seniors are going to pay additional charges for health care, they would rather have protection against long-term-care costs than the benefits provided through the MCCA. Many seniors asserted this view and Congress listened.

Medicare's Limitations

From the older consumer's point of view, Medicare is a double-edged sword—it is both indispensable and limited. Medicare was originally designed to cover only the costs of acute care and not chronic conditions. Most importantly, Medicare does not cover the costs of long-term or "custodial care" either at home or in a nursing home. Custodial care includes help in such activities as walking or getting in and out of bed.

In 1988 approximately 6.9 million older Americans were in need of such care. According to the American Association of Retired Persons (AARP), expenses for long-term care are the major catastrophic health-care expense for older Americans. For instance, about one-third of the elderly who spend any time in a nursing home become poor. Similarly, about half of single elderly people who live alone become impoverished when home care is provided for only five days a week for 26 weeks.

Other major limitations of Medicare are its complexity and limited reimbursement. Medicare's benefit structure and payment mechanisms are baffling to the best and brightest. A nationwide survey by AARP found that the majority of persons age 65 and older did not know what services Medicare actually covered.

Medicare works on a principle of cost sharing. In other words, it *shares* the costs with recipients, it *does not pay all of the costs itself*. As such, Medicare picks up the tab for only about 40 percent of all health care for its recipients.

Medicare also has specific, often confusing, standards for the services it does cover, and it does not pay for care that is not considered "reasonable and necessary" *even if a physician ordered such care.* For example, Medicare does not cover preventive health care. In other words, Medicare does *not* pay to help beneficiaries steer clear of disease, but *does* pay if disease strikes. Medicare will also not pay for routine examinations and such necessities as eyeglasses, hearing aids, or dentures. In addition, Medicare will not pay in the following circumstances: if a beneficiary visits a doctor more than is absolutely necessary, if a doctor places a beneficiary in a hospital when the kind of care received could be provided somewhere else, or when a stay in a hospital or skilled nursing facility is no longer needed.

Eligibility for Medicare

A Medicare card is automatically mailed to Social Security and Railroad Retirement beneficiaries three months before their sixty-fifth birthday. (See Figure 1.1.) The card is the ticket to obtaining services by Medicare-approved suppliers. Recipients only need to complete the card and return it to Social Security if they *don't* want Part B benefits for which there *is a charge.* All

HEALTH **INSURANCE**

SOCIAL SECURITY ACT

NAME OF BENEFICIARY JENNIFER SMITH

CLAIM NUMBER 123-45-6789 A   SEX F

IS ENTITLED TO   EFFECTIVE DATE
HOSPITAL INSURANCE   1-1-90
MEDICAL INSURANCE   1-1-90
SIGN HERE ➡ *Jennifer Smith*

Figure 1.1   Sample of a Medicare Card.

Social Security and Railroad Retirement beneficiaries are entitled to receive Part A for which there *is no charge*. Individuals who delay enrollment in Part B can sign up at a later date, but they will have to pay a substantial penalty that increases with time.

Anyone not eligible for Medicare through Social Security or Railroad Retirement can apply to purchase Medicare coverage through paying a monthly premium. (See Figure 1.2.) Medicare is also available to persons under age 65 who have been receiving cash disability benefits from Social Security for at least two years and to persons with permanent kidney failure who are getting monthly benefits under Social Security or the Railroad Retirement system or have worked long enough in federal employment. In addition, under certain conditions the spouse, divorced spouse, widow or widower, or dependent parents of a qualified person may qualify for Medicare. *A spouse who is younger than age 65 is not eligible for Medicare.*

Medicare eligibility can end for beneficiaries under the following circumstances:

If a beneficiary who is covered under the spouse's work record is divorced before a marriage has lasted for 10 years

If a beneficiary does not pay the premiums

If a beneficiary voluntarily cancels

If a beneficiary is receiving coverage because of a disability and he or she recovers before reaching age 65

If a beneficiary is receiving coverage because of permanent kidney failure, protection ends 12 months after the month maintenance dialysis treatment stops or 36 months after the month of a successful kidney transplant

Medicare's Disability Benefits

Regardless of age, individuals who meet certain tests for disability can receive Medicare benefits. Disabled persons who have received monthly benefits from Social Security's disability program for 24 months automatically receive Medicare Part A. Those who want to receive Medicare Part B must enroll and pay

DEPARTMENT OF HEALTH AND HUMAN SERVICES
HEALTH CARE FINANCING ADMINISTRATION

Form Approved
OMB No. 0938-0251

(Do not write in this space)

APPLICATION FOR HOSPITAL INSURANCE

(This application form may also be used to
enroll in Supplementary Medical Insurance)

I apply for entitlement to Medicare's hospital insurance under Part A of title XVIII of the Social Security Act, as presently amended, and for any cash benefits to which I may be entitled under title II of that Act.

1.	(a) Print your name ——————➤	(First name, middle initial, last name)
	(b) Enter your sex (check one) ——————➤	☐ Male ☐ Female
	(c) Enter your Social Security Number ——➤	_ _ _ / _ _ / _ _ _ _
2.	Enter your name at birth if different from item 1 ——————➤	
3.	(a) Enter your date of birth (Month,day,year) ——➤	
	(b) Enter name of State or foreign country where you were born ➤ If you have already submitted a public or religious record of your birth made before you were age 5, go on to item 4)	
	(c) Was a public record of your birth made before you were age 5?	☐ Yes ☐ No ☐ Unknown
	(d) Was a religious record of your birth made before you were age 5?	☐ Yes ☐ No ☐ Unknown
4.	(a) Have you (or has someone on your behalf) ever filed an application for social security benefits, a period of disability under social security, supplemental security income, or hospital or medical insurance under Medicare? ——————➤	☐ Yes ☐ No If "Yes," answer (If "No," go on (b) and (c).) to item 5.)
	(b) Enter name of person on whose social security record you filed other application. ——————➤	
	(c) Enter Social Security Number of person named in (b). (If unknown, so indicate) ——————➤	_ _ _ / _ _ / _ _ _ _
5.	(a) Were you in the active military or naval service (including Reserve or National Guard active duty or active duty for training) after September 7, 1939? ——————➤	☐ Yes ☐ No If "Yes," answer (If "No," go on (b) and (c).) to item 6)
	(b) Enter dates of service ——————➤	From: (Month, year) To: (Month, year)
	(c) Have you ever been (or will you be) eligible for a monthly benefit from a military or civilian Federal agency? (Include Veterans Administration benefits only if you waived military retirement pay) ➤	☐ Yes ☐ No
6.	Did you work in the railroad industry any time on or after January 1, 1937? ——————➤	☐ Yes ☐ No

Form HCFA-18 F5 (3-80) Previous editions of this form are obsolete   Page 1   (Over)

Figure 1.2   Application To Purchase Medicare Coverage. Form HCFA-18 F5.

12

Figure 1.2 (continued)

7.	(a) Have you ever engaged in work that was covered under the social security system of a country other than the United States? ➡	☐ Yes ☐ No
	(b) If "Yes," list the country(ies). ➡	
8.	(a) How much were your total earnings last year? ➡ *(If none, write "None")*	Earnings $
	(b) How much do you expect your total earnings to be this year? ➡ *(If none, write "None")*	Earnings $
9.	Are you a resident of the United States? ➡ *(To reside in a place means to make a home there.)*	☐ Yes ☐ No
10.	(a) Are you a citizen of the United States? ➡ *(If "Yes," go on to item 11.) (If "No," answer (b) and (c) below.)*	☐ Yes ☐ No
	(b) Are you lawfully admitted for permanent residence in the United States? ➡	☐ Yes ☐ No

(c) Enter below the information requested about your place of residence in the last 5 years:

ADDRESS AT WHICH YOU RESIDED IN THE LAST 5 YEARS (Begin with the most recent address. Show actual date residence began even if that is prior to the last 5 years.)	DATE RESIDENCE BEGAN			DATE RESIDENCE ENDED		
	Month	Day	Year	Month	Day	Year

(If you need more space, use the "Remarks" space on the third page or another sheet of paper)

| 11. | Are you currently married? ➡ | ☐ Yes ☐ No |
| | *(If "Yes," give the following information about your current marriage.) (If "No," go on to item 12.)* | |

YOUR CURRENT MARRIAGE

To whom married *(Enter your wife's maiden name or your husband's name)*	When *(Month, day, year)*
Spouse's date of birth (or age)	Spouse's Social Security Number *(If none or unknown, so indicate)* __ __ __ / __ __ / __ __ __ __

12. If you had a previous marriage and your spouse died, OR if you had a previous marriage which lasted 10 or more years, give the following information. *(If you had no previous marriage(s), enter "NONE.")*

YOUR PREVIOUS MARRIAGE

To whom married *(Enter your wife's maiden name or your husband's name).*	When *(Month, day, year)*
Spouse's date of birth (or age)	Spouse's Social Security Number *(If none or unknown, so indicate)* __ __ __ / __ __ / __ __ __ __
If spouse deceased, give date of death ➡	

(Use "Remarks" space on page 3 for information about any other marriages.)

Figure 1.2   (continued)

13.	Is or was your spouse a railroad worker, railroad retirement pensioner, or a railroad retirement annuitant? ——————————————————►	☐ Yes	☐ No
14.	(a) Were you or your spouse a civilian employee of the Federal Government after June 1960? ——————————————► (If "Yes," answer (b).) (If "No," omit (b), (c), and (d).)	☐ Yes	☐ No
	(b) Are you or your spouse now covered under a medical insurance plan provided by the Federal Employees Health Benefits Act of 1959?► *(If "Yes," omit (c) and (d).) (If "No," answer (c).)*	☐ Yes	☐ No
	(c) Are you **and** your spouse barred from coverage under the above Act because your Federal employment, or your spouse's was not long enough? ————————————————► *(If "Yes," omit (d) and explain in "Remarks" below.) (If "No," answer (d).)*	☐ Yes	☐ No
	(d) Were either you or your spouse an employee of the Federal Government after February 15, 1965? ————————►	☐ Yes	☐ No

Remarks:

_____

_____

_____

_____

_____

_____

15.	If you are found to be otherwise ineligible for hospital insurance under Medicare, do you wish to enroll for hospital insurance on a monthly premium basis (in addition to the monthly premium for supplementary medical insurance)?—————————————————————► *(If "Yes," you MUST also sign up for medical insurance.)*	☐ Yes	☐ No

INFORMATION ON MEDICAL INSURANCE UNDER MEDICARE

Medical insurance under Medicare helps pay your doctor bills. It also helps pay for a number of other medical items and services not covered under the hospital insurance part of Medicare.

If you sign up for medical insurance, you must pay a premium for each month you have this protection. If you get monthly social security, railroad retirement, or civil service benefits, your premium will be deducted from your benefit check, If you get none of these benefits, you will be notified how to pay your premium.

The Federal Government contributes to the cost of your insurance. The amount of your premium and the Government's payment are based on the cost of services covered by medical insurance. The Government also makes additional payments when necessary to meet the full cost of the program. (Currently, the Government pays about two-thirds of the cost of this program.) You will get advance notice if there is any change in your premium amount.

If you have questions or would like a leaflet on medical insurance, call any Social Security office.

| SEE OTHER SIDE TO SIGN UP FOR MEDICAL INSURANCE |

14

Figure 1.2 (continued)

If you become entitled to hospital insurance as a result of this application, you will be enrolled for medical insurance automatically unless you indicate below that you do not want this protection. If you decline to enroll now, you can get medical insurance protection later only if you sign up for it during specified enrollment periods. Your protection may then be delayed and you may have to pay a higher premium when you decide to sign up.

The date your medical insurance begins and the amount of the premium you must pay depend on the month you file this application with the Social Security Administration. Any social security office will be glad to explain the rules regarding enrollment to you.

16.	DO YOU WISH TO ENROLL FOR SUPPLEMENTARY MEDICAL IN-SURANCE? ⟶ *(If "Yes," answer question 17.)*	☐ Yes ☐ No ☐ Currently Enrolled
17.	Are you or your spouse receiving an annuity under the Federal Civil Service Retirement Act or other law administered by the Office of Personnel Management ? ⟶	☐ Yes ☐ No
		Your No.
	(If "Yes," enter Civil Service annuity number here. Include the prefix "CSA" for annuitant, "CSF" for survivor.)	Spouse's No.
	If you entered your spouse's number, is he (she) enrolled for supplementary medical insurance under social security? ⟶	☐ Yes⁓ ☐ No

I know that anyone who makes or causes to be made a false statement or representation of material fact in an application or for use in determining a right to payment under the Social Security Act commits a crime punishable under Federal law by fine, imprisonment or both. I affirm that all information I have given in this document is true.

SIGNATURE OF APPLICANT	Date *(Month, day, year)*
Signature *(First name, middle initial, last name) (Write in ink)* **SIGN HERE** ▶	Telephone Number(s) at which you may be contacted during the day

Mailing Address *(Number and street, Apt. No., P.O. Box, or Rural Route)*

City and State	ZIP Code	Enter Name of County (if any) in which you now live

Witnesses are required ONLY if this application has been signed by mark (X) above. If signed by mark (X), two witnesses to the signing who know the applicant must sign below, giving their full addresses.

1. Signature of Witness	2. Signature of Witness
Address *(Number and street, City, State, and ZIP Code)*	Address *(Number and street, City, State, and ZIP Code)*

Form HCFA-18 F5 (3-80) Page 4

Figure 1.2   (continued)

A REMINDER TO APPLICANTS FOR THE SOCIAL SECURITY HOSPITAL INSURANCE

NAME OF PERSON TO CONTACT ABOUT YOUR CLAIM	SSA OFFICE	DATE
TELEPHONE NO.		

RECEIPT FOR YOUR CLAIM

Your application for the hospital insurance has been received and will be processed as quickly as possible.

You should hear from us within   days after you have given us all the information we requested. Some claims may take longer if additional information is needed.

In the meantime, if you change your mailing address, you should report the change.

Always give us your claim number when writing or telephoning about your claim.

If you have any questions about your claim, we will be glad to help you.

CLAIMANT	SOCIAL SECURITY CLAIM NUMBER

COLLECTION AND USE OF INFORMATION FROM YOUR APPLICATION — PRIVACY ACT NOTICE

PRIVACY ACT NOTICE: The Social Security Administration (SSA) is authorized to collect the information on this form under sections 226 and 1818 of the Social Security Act, as amended (42 U.S.C. 426 and 1395-17) and section 103 of Public Law 89-97. The information on this form is needed to enable social security and the Health Care Financing Administration (HCFA) to determine if you and your dependents may be entitled to hospital and/or medical insurance coverage and/or monthly benefits. While you do not have to furnish the information requested on this form to social security, no benefits or hospital or medical insurance can be provided until an application has been received by a social security office. Failure to provide all or part of the information requested could prevent an accurate and timely decision on your claim or your dependent's claim, and could result in the loss of some benefits or hospital or medical insurance. Although the infor-

mation you furnish on this form is almost never used for any other purpose than stated above, there is a possibility that for the administration of the social security or HCFA programs or for the administration of programs requiring coordination with SSA or HCFA, information may be disclosed to another person or to another governmental agency as follows: 1) to enable a third party or an agency to assist social security or HCFA in establishing rights to social security benefits and/or hospital or medical insurance coverage; 2) to comply with Federal laws requiring the release of information from social security and HCFA records (e.g., to the General Accounting Office and the Veterans Administration); and 3) to facilitate statistical research and audit activities necessary to assure the integrity and improvement of the social security and HCFA programs (e.g., to the Bureau of the Census and private concerns under contract to social security and HCFA).

a monthly premium. Workers who are insured under Social Security and members of their families who need dialysis treatment or a kidney transplant because of permanent kidney failure also are eligible for Medicare.

Social Security periodically reviews disability cases to determine whether recipients of benefits have improved and, therefore, are ineligible for benefits. Generally, benefits are stopped if a Social Security review shows that the impairment that caused the disability has medically improved. After a review Social Security will notify the individual in writing, and the disabled person has 60 days to file an appeal.

Disabled persons who want to continue to work can, under limited circumstances, still receive Medicare. Local Social Security offices provide information on disability benefits.

Medicare Assistance Programs

The federal government has designated regional Health Care Financing Administration (HCFA) and local Social Security offices as the places to go for help on Medicare and related problems. However, in reality, Social Security offices only take applications for Medicare, and the staff is generally not well informed about the program. Social Security and HCFA offices are also very hard to reach by phone.

Many communities now offer programs that help Medicare recipients understand their benefits. The Medicare Medicaid Assistance Program (MMAP), sponsored by the American Association of Retired Persons, provides counseling on Medicare and supplemental health insurance. MMAP is in most states across the country. In addition, California, Colorado, Connecticut, Illinois, Massachusetts, Missouri, New Jersey, North Carolina, Washington, Wisconsin, and other states provide health-insurance counseling programs for seniors. Most of these programs are run by well-trained volunteers who provide information services for Medicare recipients to help them understand their benefits. Many also offer assistance in filing claims. In addition, HCFA is now offering Medicare training programs for seniors across the country, and local aging offices or legal-service programs should know if such programs are available in their area.

Table 1.1   Medicare Benefits and Costs

PART A	PART B
MAJOR BENEFITS	
Inpatient Hospital Care	Doctors' Services
Skilled-Nursing Facility Care (under limited circumstances)	Outpatient Services
	Medical Equipment
Home Health Care (under limited circumstances)	Physical Therapy
	Laboratory Tests
Hospice Care	Home Health Care (under limited circumstances)
	Hospice Care
MAJOR COSTS	
No Premium	Monthly Premium ($28.60 in 1990)
Inpatient Hospital Deductible per Benefit Period ($592 in 1990)	Annual Deductible
Coinsurance for Days 61–90 of Hospitalization ($148 in 1990)	20 Percent Coinsurance plus Any Excess Charge for Unassigned Claims
Coinsurance for Days 21–100 in a Nursing Home ($74 in 1990)	Uncovered Services
Uncovered Services	

The Medicare Handbook

Once a year the HCFA publishes an important tool to understanding the Medicare program: *The Medicare Handbook*. The
handbook provides details on the program, and Medicare beneficiaries automatically receive a copy when they enroll. However,
updated copies are *not* sent to beneficiaries every year. It is
important for beneficiaries to get each year's edition of the handbook from a Social Security office in order to keep up on changes
in benefits.

Medicare's Two Parts

As previously mentioned, Medicare is a two-part system. Parts A
and B of Medicare work together to provide a single comprehensive insurance program. Medicare's two parts are roughly based
on the division in the medical community between hospitals and
physicians. In spite of the fact that in a hospital patient care is
provided by physicians, few physicians actually work for hospitals. Most are independent business people. Therefore, patients

receive separate bills from the hospitals and the doctors. Similarly, Medicare has two parts: A, which is the hospitalization program; and B, which pays doctors' bills and outpatient expenses. Details of these programs follow in the next two chapters.

THINGS TO REMEMBER

Medicare beneficiaries should be sure when choosing health providers that they are approved for Medicare payments. Medicare will not pay for care received from nonparticipating (not Medicare-approved) hospitals, skilled-nursing facilities, home health agencies, or hospices. There is one exception: Medicare will pay if the individual has been sent to a nonparticipating hospital in an emergency, and if the hospital is the closest one equipped to handle the problem. (See Table 1.1 for a quick synopsis of Part A and Part B benefits.)

Chapter 2

Medicare Part A

- Medicare Part A will help pay for services qualified individuals receive in a hospital, skilled-nursing facility, home health agency, or hospice program.

- Medicare will pay for the first 60 days of inpatient hospital care per "spell of illness" after the patient pays a deductible ($592 in 1990).

- If a patient is hospitalized for more than 60 days, coinsurance is required for days 61 through 90 ($148 per day in 1990).

- Except in limited circumstances, Medicare does not help pay for hospital and related services outside of the United States.

- Medicare coverage of nursing homes is very limited, paying for less than 2 percent of all nursing-home costs for the elderly.

- If an individual requires inpatient, *daily* skilled nursing or rehabilitation *after a hospital stay,* Medicare will cover all of the charges for the first 20 days in a skilled nursing facility. It will also pay *part* of the charges for another 80 days, but the older patient must pay coinsurance ($74 per day in 1990).

- For those who qualify, Medicare will cover limited home health care services for an unlimited number of days.

- Medicare will pay for 210 days of hospice care for those who qualify.

- Beneficiaries do not have to send Medicare bills for care received from a *Medicare-approved* hospital, skilled-nursing facility, home health agency, or hospice. Medicare pays benefits directly to the hospital or other facility.

Introduction

Medicare Part A helps to pay for hospital room-and-board costs and three newer, less-expensive alternatives to hospitals— skilled-nursing facilities, home health care, and hospice care. Services of a physician while a beneficiary is in a Part A facility are covered under Medicare Part B.

Inpatient Hospital Care

Hospitals provide the backdrops and props for the most important events in life—birth and death. They are the centers where the medical profession treats individuals with acute illnesses or serious injuries. The germ of today's modern hospital system began 4,000 years before Christ when the forerunners of medical schools were the temples of Saturn in ancient Egypt. The first U.S. hospitals were almshouses for the homeless and poor and pesthouses for isolating people with contagious diseases. The purpose of both was to protect society from undesirable and diseased residents—there was no serious attempt to provide care for patients. Almshouses and pesthouses were common in big cities in the mid-eighteenth century, and eventually, many developed separate infirmaries that did more than just protect the public from the unwanted. By the mid-nineteenth century large hospitals began to flourish; the most notable of these were Bellevue Hospital in New York City and General Hospital in Boston.

In this century hospitals have become the pulse of the medical-care system, as well as a major force in the U.S. economy. Hospitals are the second- or third-largest employer in the United

States. Expenditures for hospitals are the largest component of national-health expenditures, representing 39 percent of total national-health spending in 1987. And the Health Care Financing Administration (HCFA) projects that in 1990 expenditures for hospitals will account for 54 percent of Medicare benefit payments.

There are 7,000 hospitals in the United States—6,715 of which were Medicare certified in 1988. They include numerous variations on the basic theme of caring for the sick and injured. Hospitals can be small (50 to 200 beds), midsized (200 to 500 beds), or large (more than 500 beds). Hospitals can be not-for-profit, investor owned, or public. They are teaching or nonteaching. The majority are general hospitals treating the full range of illnesses and injuries. However, some will treat only patients with specific problems, such as respiratory illnesses, mental illness, or cancer. There are also special hospitals for the military and veterans. Finally, there are medical centers and community hospitals. The former are usually best for serious complicated problems and the latter when routine care is needed and/or a more personal touch is desired.

About one out of three older adults is hospitalized annually. Most are admitted for acute episodes of chronic conditions. The most common admissions are for diseases of the circulatory system (including heart disease), digestive diseases, respiratory diseases (including pneumonia), and neoplasms. On average there are about four diagnoses per older person admitted to a hospital, compared to two for younger persons.

The cost of hospitalization for older persons was $2,248 per capita in 1987, with Medicare paying 70 percent of this amount. Estimates for 1990 are that Medicare will spend $58.6 billion on inpatient hospital services, which will take up more than half (54 percent) of the entire Medicare budget.

Medicare's Rules for Qualifying for Inpatient Hospital Services

Medicare will help pay for inpatient hospital services if all of the following conditions are met:

1. A physician prescribes inpatient hospital care for the treatment of an illness or injury

2. The beneficiary requires and receives the kind of care that can only be provided in a hospital

3. The hospital is participating in Medicare

4. The Utilization Review Committee (URC) of the hospital or the Peer Review Organization (PRO) does not disapprove the stay

Medicare Coverage

Medicare Part A pays for the first 60 days of a semiprivate room, meals, regular nursing, drugs, lab tests, X rays and other radiology services, special-care units, medical supplies, blood (after the first three pints), rehabilitation, appliances, operating- and recovery-room costs, and supplies in the hospital after the patient pays a deductible ($592 in 1990). (Medicare will also pay for a private hospital room when medically necessary.) In addition, if a patient is hospitalized for an additional 30 days, Medicare will pay part of the expenses, but coinsurance is required for days 61 through 90 ($148 per day in 1990).

Except in limited circumstances, Medicare does not help pay for hospital and related services outside of the United States. It will pay in Canadian and Mexican hospitals only at the following times:

When a beneficiary is in the United States and an emergency occurs, and a Canadian or Mexican hospital is closer than the nearest U.S. hospital that can provide emergency services

When a beneficiary lives in the United States, and a Canadian or Mexican hospital is closer to home than the nearest U.S. hospital

When a beneficiary is in Canada, traveling on a direct route between Alaska and another state, and an emergency occurs

If a beneficiary is in a Canadian or Mexican hospital under these circumstances he or she must submit the hospital bills, which is not the case in U.S. hospitals. To protect themselves, beneficiaries who plan to travel overseas may want to purchase short-term health insurance for travel.

Costs to Beneficiaries

Medicare coverage in a hospital is based on "benefit periods" or "spells of illness," which are designated periods of time in which a Medicare patient may receive coverage. Each benefit period for hospital coverage begins the first day that the patient enters the hospital and lasts for 90 days. Beneficiaries must pay deductibles and coinsurance for each benefit period. The hospital deductible is an initial amount the beneficiary must pay in each benefit period before Medicare will pay its share. Coinsurance is a dollar amount that the beneficiary must pay for each day of care between days 61 and 90 in each benefit period.

Medicare patients must also cover the costs of extras, such as televisions and telephones, private-duty nurses, a private room, and, with some exceptions, care in hospitals outside the United States. Except under limited circumstances, beneficiaries will have to pay for hospitalization outside of the United States.

There is a limited safety valve for the small number of Medicare hospital patients who require extended inpatient care. Each Medicare beneficiary receives a lifetime reserve of 60 days of hospital coverage, which can be used if hospitalization is required beyond a 90-day benefit period. Medicare patients pay a daily coinsurance for each reserve day used. Medicare pays for no more than 190 days of inpatient care in a psychiatric hospital in a beneficiary's lifetime.

THINGS TO REMEMBER

An individual cannot just check himself or herself into a hospital. Hospitals have strict utilization review guidelines for Medicare patients, limiting who is admitted and how long they can stay. A physician must prescribe inpatient hospital care. However, even then, a hospital stay by a Medicare patient can be disapproved by the hospital's Utilization Review Committee or the state Peer Review Organization.

When hospitalized, Medicare recipients receive important notices titled "An Important Message from Medicare." (See Figure 2.1.) Among other things, the notice spells out the right of

AN IMPORTANT MESSAGE FROM MEDICARE

YOUR RIGHTS WHILE YOU ARE A MEDICARE HOSPITAL PATIENT

- You have the right to receive all the hospital care that is necessary for the proper diagnosis and treatment of your illness or injury. According to Federal law, **your discharge date must be determined solely by your medical needs**, not by "DRGs" or Medicare payments.

- You have the right to be fully informed about decisions affecting your Medicare coverage and payment for your hospital stay and for any post-hospital services.

- You have the right to request a review by a Peer Organization of any written Notice of Noncoverage that you receive from the hospital stating that Medicare will no longer pay for your hospital care. Peer Review Organizations (PROs) are groups of doctors who are paid by the Federal Government to review medical necessity, appropriateness and quality of hospital treatment furnished to Medicare patients. The phone number and address of the PRO for this area is:

Colorado Foundation for Medical Care
6825 East Tennessee Avenue
Building 2, Suite 400
PO Box 17300
Denver, Colorado 80127   Telephone: (303) 321-8642

TALK TO YOUR DOCTOR ABOUT YOUR STAY IN THE HOSPITAL

You and your doctor know more about your condition and your health needs than anyone else. Decisions about your medical treatment should be made between you and your doctor. **If you have any questions about your medical treatment, your need for continued hospital care, your discharge, or your need for possible post-hospital care, don't hesitate to ask your doctor.** The hospital's patient representative or social worker will also help you with your questions and concerns about hospital services.

IF YOU THINK YOU ARE BEING ASKED TO LEAVE THE HOSPITAL TOO SOON

- Ask a hospital representative for a written notice of explanation immediately, if you have not already received one. This notice is called a "Notice of Noncoverage." You must have this Notice of Noncoverage if you wish to exercise your right to request a review by the PRO.

- The Notice of Noncoverage will state either that your doctor or the PRO agrees with the hospital's decision that Medicare will no longer pay for your hospital care.

  + If the hospital and your doctor agree, the PRO does not review your case before a Notice of Noncoverage is issued. But the PRO will respond to your request for a review of your Notice of Noncoverage and seek your opinion. You cannot be made to pay for your hospital care until the PRO makes its decision, if you request the review by noon of the first work day after you receive the Notice of Noncoverage.

  + If the hospital and your doctor disagree, the hospital may request the PRO to review your case. If it does make such a request, the hospital is required to send you a notice to that effect. In this situation the PRO must agree with the hospital or the hospital cannot issue a Notice of Noncoverage but since the PRO has already reviewed your case once, you may have to pay for **at least one day of hospital care** before the PRO completes this reconsideration.

IF YOU DO NOT REQUEST A REVIEW, THE HOSPITAL MAY BILL YOU FOR ALL THE COSTS OF YOUR STAY BEGINNING WITH THE THIRD DAY AFTER YOU RECEIVE THE NOTICE OF NONCOVERAGE. THE HOSPITAL, HOWEVER, CANNOT CHARGE YOU FOR CARE UNLESS IT PROVIDES YOU WITH A NOTICE OF NONCOVERAGE.

Figure 2.1   An Important Message from Medicare.

Figure 2.1   (continued)

HOW TO REQUEST A REVIEW OF THE NOTICE OF NONCOVERAGE

- If the Notice of Noncoverage states that your **physician agrees** with the hospital's decision:

  + You must make your request for review to the PRO by **noon of the first work day** after you receive the Notice of Noncoverage by contacting the PRO by phone or in writing.

  + The PRO must ask for your views about your case before making its decision. The PRO will inform you by phone and in writing of its decision on the review.

  + If the PRO agrees with the Notice of Noncoverage, you may be billed for all costs of your stay beginning at noon of the day **after** you receive the PRO's decision.

  + Thus, you will **not** be responsible for the cost of hospital care before you receive the PRO's decision.

- If the Notice of Noncoverage states that the **PRO agrees** with the hospital's decision:

  + You should make your request for reconsideration to the PRO **immediately** upon receipt of the Notice of Noncoverage by contacting the PRO by phone or in writing.

  + The PRO can take up to three working days from receipt of your request to complete the review. The PRO will inform you in writing of its decision on the review.

  + Since the PRO has already reviewed your case once, prior to the issuance of the Notice on Noncoverage, the hospital is permitted to begin billing you for the cost of your stay beginning with the third calendar day after you receive your Notice of Noncoverage, **even if the PRO has not completed its review.**

  + Thus, if the PRO continues to agree with the Notice of Nonccoverage, you **may have to pay for at least one day of hospital care.**

NOTE: The process described above is called "immediate review." If you miss the deadline for this immediate review while you are in the hospital, you may still request a review of Medicare's decision to no longer pay for your care at any point during your hospital stay or after you have left the hospital. The Notice of Noncoverage will tell you how to request this review.

POST-HOSPITAL CARE

When your doctor determines that you no longer need all the specialized services provided in a hospital, but you still require medical care, he or she may discharge you to a skilled nursing facility or home care. The discharge planner at the hospital will help arrange for the services you may need after your discharge. Medicare and supplemental insurance policies have limited coverage for skilled nursing facility care and home health care. Therefore, you should find out which services will or will not be covered and how payment will be made. Consult with your doctor, hospital discharge planner, patient representative and your family in making preparations for care after you leave the hospital. **Don't hesitate to ask questions.**

ACKNOWLEDGEMENT OF RECEIPT—My signature only acknowledges my receipt of this Message from   and does not waive any of my rights to request a review or make me liable for any payment.

_____   _____
Signature of beneficiary or person acting on behalf of beneficiary   Date

Patient Name _____ Hospital Number _____

Medicare patients to receive all the hospital care that is necessary for the proper diagnosis and treatment of the illness or injury. These rights are particularly important under Medicare's prospective payment system. (For important information about hospital patient rights, see Chapter 5.)

Skilled-Nursing-Facility (SNF) Care

Nursing homes in the United States date back to the early American boardinghouses or hotels, whose clients were predominantly retired and aged, as well as the almshouses and pesthouses of the nineteenth and twentieth centuries. The first homes specifically designated for the elderly were sponsored by voluntary and religious organizations. In the 1940s and 1950s the need for nursing homes increased as the result of two forces: (1) the numbers of elderly burgeoned, and (2) they also had an increasing ability to pay for care through cash payments from Social Security and Old Age Assistance, the precursor of the Supplemental Security Income (SSI). In response to the demand for nursing homes, from the 1950s to the mid-1960s government programs provided loans and mortgage insurance for building facilities, resulting in an increased supply. By 1980 there were more than 24,121 nursing homes. In 1988, 7,379 skilled-nursing homes were Medicare certified.

Nursing homes care for people with physical limitations by isolating them from the community in institutional settings. The term *nursing home* refers to facilities that range from small "Mom and Pop" homes to large government-run facilities with 1,000 or more beds. As a general rule the term *home* in nursing home is a misnomer. Nursing home administration is based on the same medical model that dominates the hospital industry. Nursing homes are institutions, and their atmosphere is representative of all the name implies.

Only about 5 percent of the older population are in nursing homes at any one point in time. However, it has been estimated that one in five persons 65 and older will enter a nursing home at some point before they die. In 1985, 1.3 million older Americans were in nursing homes. Estimates for annual expenses for individuals in nursing homes range from $22,000 to $50,000. The cost of nursing-home care for older persons was $1,085 per capita in 1987.

Medicare coverage of nursing homes is very limited. Medicare pays less than 2 percent of total nursing-home costs for individuals and payments for skilled-nursing homes make up only 1 percent of the Medicare budget. (For more information about nursing homes, see Chapter 7.)

Medicare Rules for Qualifying for SNF Coverage

Medicare will cover the expenses for only one specific type of facility, the skilled-nursing facility (SNF). An SNF is a specially qualified facility that has the staff and equipment to provide skilled-nursing care or rehabilitation services and other related services. If an individual requires inpatient, *daily* skilled nursing or rehabilitation, Medicare will pay for up to 100 days of care per benefit period. Prior hospitalization for at least three continuous days is required.

As a general rule, a number of factors determine whether Medicare will cover skilled-nursing care: (1) if the patient was hospitalized for three days in a row, not counting the day of discharge, (2) if the patient was transferred to the SNF for care of the same condition that was treated in the hospital, (3) if the patient is admitted to the SNF within a short time after leaving the hospital (usually 30 days), (4) if a doctor certifies that *daily* care is required, and (5) if the stay is not disapproved by the facility's Utilization Review Committee or Peer Review Organization. There are several nuances to the daily rule. They are the following:

> The resident does not need to receive the same service every day
>
> If a needed service is not available on weekends, the reimbursement will not be denied
>
> If the resident's physician determines that there should be a short break from services, the reimbursement will not be denied

Medicare Coverage

Part A's skilled-nursing-facility benefit pays for a semiprivate room, meals, regular nursing, rehabilitation, drugs, blood, supplies, and appliances. "Swing beds" in hospitals that can be used either as a hospital or skilled-nursing bed can qualify as long as they are certified by Medicare.

Costs to Beneficiaries

Keeping in mind that Medicare's guidelines for SNF coverage are very strict and many beneficiaries may have to cover all of their own costs, those who qualify may receive help with 100 days of coverage per benefit period. Medicare's current SNF coverage works on the same principle of benefit periods that is applicable to its hospital coverage. However, SNF benefit periods run for 100 days, require coinsurance from days 21 through 100 ($74 in 1990), and there are no reserve days.

In 1987 the interim cost of a day in a Medicare SNF was $73. Medicare does not cover the cost of personal convenience items, private-duty nurses, extra charges for a private room, and custodial-nursing services provided to persons with chronic, long-term illnesses or disabilities. Beneficiaries do not have to cover the full costs of doctors' visits and therapy that are covered by Medicare Part B.

As previously mentioned, older adults have to cover the costs of intermediate or custodial care, commonly referred to as long-term care. *Medicare does not cover these costs under any circumstances.*

THINGS TO REMEMBER

When selecting nursing homes, beneficiaries should be sure that the facility is a Medicare-certified skilled-nursing facility. Many nursing homes are not skilled-nursing facilities and not all skilled-nursing facilities are Medicare certified. If a facility does not give a clear answer in this regard, beneficiaries should be suspicious and check with the state Medicare intermediary. *Medicare recipients should also remember that there are specific guidelines for Medicare coverage of SNFs; they cannot just check into an SNF and expect Medicare to pay for the care.* Placement in an SNF should be discussed carefully with the patient's doctor.

Because of Medicare's narrow guidelines for paying for skilled-nursing homes, certified facilities often have trouble getting reimbursed for residents. And under a rule called a "waiver of liability" the facility administrators may be concerned that they will have to pick up the costs if Medicare turns them down. (If they do not submit a bill, then the beneficiary is responsible, not the facility.) Residents may be told by a facility that they will have to pay for their stays themselves and that the facility is not going to submit a bill to Medicare. However, Medicare patients have a right to demand that the Medicare-certified facility send the claim in to Medicare. This is called a demand or no-payment billing, which tells Medicare that the facility expects no payment from Medicare, but the beneficiary has "demanded" submission of the claim. *In most cases, beneficiaries should exercise this right. If a claim has not been sent in, the beneficiary cannot appeal the case.* (For more information on SNF claims, see Chapter 5.)

Home Health Care

In-home services were first offered by welfare agencies in the early 1900s when private charities provided homemakers to care for children with sick mothers. Organized home health care began with voluntary agencies in big cities, which grew into the well-known, highly regarded Visiting Nurse Association. Hospital-based services were started by Montefiore Hospital in New York City in the late 1940s.

Home health care can range from such high-tech services as computerized electrical-impulse devices that allow paralyzed people to walk, to a helping hand in getting in and out of bed. However, *the Medicare definition of home health care is specific and limiting.* It refers to care provided in the person's home by a registered nurse or related professional or aide under the supervision of a physician. Congress established the Medicare home health care benefit as a less extensive and less costly alternative to hospital inpatient care. Medicare interprets these guidelines very narrowly, although there is considerable variation according to region.

The Medicare home health benefit takes up only a small part of the total Medicare budget—4 percent of total outlays. Nevertheless, until recently the home health benefit was the fastest growing Medicare program. From 1981 to 1987 the number of home-care agencies participating in the Medicare program increased from 3,000 to 5,900. The HCFA projected that in 1989 Medicare would spend $2.9 billion on home health care, with an average of 1,318 visits per 1,000 Medicare enrollees at an average cost of $69 per visit. Within the next five years the total cost to Medicare is expected to rise by 63 percent to $5.2 billion, based on an average of 1,365 visits per 1,000 enrollees and $90 per visit. (For more information on home health care, see Chapter 7.)

Medicare's Rules for Qualifying for Home Health Care Coverage

The following criteria must be met for Medicare to pay for skilled care in the home:

The individual must be homebound

The care needed must include part-time skilled-nursing care, physical therapy, or speech therapy

The physician must determine that the individual needs intermittent skilled-nursing care, physical therapy, or speech therapy

The physician must write a plan of care

The home health agency providing the service must be certified by Medicare

Even though *The Medicare Handbook* and other government publications make it sound as though these benefits are readily available, the criteria are interpreted very strictly by the intermediaries who oversee the administration of the Medicare home health care benefit, and many requests for reimbursement are turned down. For example, for the individual to receive services a physician must certify that the beneficiary is "confined" to the home. This means that he or she cannot leave the home without a wheelchair or comparable help. In the past these benefits have been repeatedly denied to beneficiaries who were able to leave their home for only short periods of time and with a great deal of assistance. (Ten percent of all claims that are denied are turned down because the patient does not meet the homebound/ intermittent category.)

Often beneficiaries who attend day care are disqualified. If home health care claims are denied because of an overly narrow interpretation of the confinement rule, they should be appealed. (For information on appeals, see Chapter 5.)

Medicare beneficiaries recently won a major victory in the courts that may improve access to home health care services for some beneficiaries. The court ruling may mean that there will be less home health care denials in the future and that some beneficiaries will be reimbursed retroactively for services that were unfairly denied. U.S. District Court Judge Stanley Sporkin ruled that the HCFA "arbitrarily" denied thousands of valid claims by unfairly restricting the part-time or intermittent definition of services. Sporkin says the denials "take away essential medical services from aged and sick people," so that many are forced into nursing homes when they could stay at home if they had the services. The suit was brought by several home-care agencies, members of Congress, the National Association of Homecare, the American Association of Retired Persons, and 17 beneficiaries who were denied home-care payments from Medicare. The court ruled that HCFA must reopen all Medicare claims denied on the part-time or intermittent basis.

Medicare usually will not pay for home health care that is for a chronic problem such as arthritis, rather than an acute problem such as recovery from a stroke. In fact, 90 percent of all claims that are denied are turned down because the services received were not medically necessary. Unless the services are highly skilled, home health care claims are likely to be denied. In general, skilled services are those that must be performed by a nurse or related professional or under their supervision. Those who need only nonskilled, supportive care are not eligible for reimbursement. However, patients receiving skilled care qualify for nonskilled care as long as the need for skilled care continues.

Medicare Coverage

If the criteria for the home health benefits are met, Medicare will cover a limited number of services. Depending on need, an unlimited number of visits are covered. There are no charges to the patient for these services.

The home health services covered under Medicare are part-time or intermittent *skilled*-nursing care, physical therapy, speech therapy, occupational therapy, part-time or intermittent services of home health aides, medical social services, and supplies and durable medical equipment.

Costs to Beneficiaries

Medicare pays the full approved costs for all covered home health visits. Beneficiaries have to pay for full-time nursing care at home, drugs and biologicals, meals delivered to the home, general housekeeping, homemaker services, shopping, and blood transfusions.

THINGS TO REMEMBER

The Medicare home health benefit is overseen by ten regional intermediaries who are responsible for administering the program. One exception is that hospital-based home health agencies are administered by the state hospital intermediaries. Home health care's intermediaries vary greatly in the ways that they interpret the Medicare home health benefit. In other words, depending on the region a beneficiary falls in, a benefit may or may not be reimbursed.

As with all Part A services, agencies bill home health care intermediaries, patients do not send bills in. However, at present it is very difficult for home health agencies to determine ahead of time if services for a particular client will be approved. Just as some SNFs are reluctant to bill Medicare for services to beneficiaries who may not qualify for Medicare reimbursement, so some home health agencies similarly will not bill Medicare intermediaries. *However, the beneficiary has a right to insist that a "demand" or "no-payment" billing be made to Medicare. Without such a billing the beneficiary cannot appeal the case if necessary.*

Hospice Care

The hospice movement originated in 1842 in France. The first hospice was opened in the United States in 1974. In 1986 Congress made the hospice benefit a permanent part of the Medicare program. Emphasizing death with dignity, hospices provide services to individuals with terminal illnesses. Hospice describes a method of care that allows the dying patient to be as comfortable as possible. The major emphasis is on regulation of drugs to provide comfort from pain while allowing the patient to be with family and friends. Hospice does not describe a particular place. The hospice method of caring for the dying can be provided in a hospital, nursing home, or at home. The Joint Commission for the Accreditation of Hospitals and Medicare have both established specific guidelines for accreditation and certification of hospices.

The majority of hospice participants are victims of cancer. In 1987 there were 417 hospices in the Medicare program, representing approximately a third of all hospices. For the period between November 1, 1983, and October 31, 1987, there were 91,475 Medicare admissions to hospices at an average cost to Medicare of $3,042 per admission and total program costs of $278 billion. The hospice benefit is minuscule compared to large Medicare programs such as inpatient hospital and physician care. Projections for 1990 are that the hospice benefit will account for less than 1 percent of total payments to beneficiaries.

Medicare's Rules for Qualifying for Hospice-Care Coverage

If an individual is *terminally ill, as certified by a physician,* they may receive up to 210 days of hospice care in a certified facility. In order to qualify for the hospice benefit the following criteria must be met:

A doctor certifies that the patient is terminally ill

A patient chooses to receive care from a hospice, instead of standard Medicare benefits for the terminal illness

Care is provided by a Medicare-certified hospice program

Medicare Coverage

Medicare will pay most of the costs of nursing, doctors, drugs (including outpatient drugs), physical therapy, speech-language pathology, occupational therapy, home health aide and home-maker services, medical social services, medical supplies and appliances, and short-term inpatient care, including limited respite care and counseling in a hospice.

Costs to Beneficiaries

With the exception of small coinsurance responsibilities for prescription drugs and respite care, Medicare pays the full approved costs for all covered hospice services. Beneficiaries must pay for treatments other than for pain relief and symptom management of the terminal illness. For example, bereavement counseling for the deceased's survivors is not covered. If a hospice patient receives treatment for a condition not related to the terminal illness, the patient still maintains all standard Medicare coverage in a hospice.

THINGS TO REMEMBER

Beneficiaries should be sure that a hospice is Medicare certified before using their services. Because of the newness of the industry, many are not.

Chapter 3

Medicare Part B

- Medicare Part B helps to pay for covered services provided by a doctor, whether it be in his or her office, in the patient's home, or in a Part A medical facility. It also covers a wide range of medical services people use when they are not patients in hospitals, such as outpatient visits to hospitals and home health visits.

- Medicare Part B was designed to pay 80 percent of the allowable charges of covered services, after payment of the deductible. Beneficiaries pay the other 20 percent, which is called the Part B coinsurance, as well as any amount above Medicare's "allowable charges."

Introduction

Medicare Part B helps to pay physicians and other medical service providers, whether in or out of the hospital. It also serves as a catchall for the wide range of medical services people use when they are not patients in hospitals, such as outpatient visits to hospitals, physical therapy, laboratory tests, medical equipment (like wheelchairs or oxygen), and home health visits. *Part B was designed to pay 80 percent of the government's approved amount of covered services, after payment of the deductible. Beneficiaries pay the other 20 percent, which is called the Part B coinsurance.* A few services such as home health benefits and second opinions for surgery are exempt from coinsurance.

The Health Services Network

Homer's poetry is thought to contain the first record of medical services. The poet described an organized and well-established health profession. Homer's heroes themselves were skilled in surgery, and there existed a well-respected professional class of medical specialists in Greece at that time. The first identified nurse was Fabiola, a patrician Roman lady, who founded a hospital in Rome with a convalescent home attached in A.D. 380.

Today the health services network is a vast system of health professionals and related workers, ranging from brain surgeons and nurses to ambulance drivers and suppliers of medical equipment. The network includes more than 550,000 physicians and 8.5 million health employees. Several million also work in related fields.

Without the help of Medicare to pay for medical services and goods, the out-of-pocket costs to the elderly would increase dramatically. According to the Health Care Financing Administration (HCFA), physician services and related personal-health care accounted for 21 percent of personal-health expenditures for the elderly in 1987, or $1,107 per capita. Medicare covered 61 percent of expenses for physician services, or $671. In turn, medical services are projected to account for 33 percent of total Medicare payments in 1990.

It is not surprising that the use of physician and related services increases with age. For example, in 1987 persons age 45 to 64 averaged 6.4 doctor contacts a year, while persons age 65 and older averaged 8.4 contacts. Since the enactment of Medicare the average number of physician contacts for the older population has increased significantly. However, use of other health services not covered by Medicare, such as dental care, is less than that of the younger population. In 1986 persons 65 and over averaged .8 visits to a dentist per year compared to 1.7 for persons 45 to 64.

The following services are covered by Medicare under Part B. It is important for beneficiaries to check this list whenever they are planning to use a particular health service to make sure that Medicare will cover its share of the costs.

Doctors' Services

Medicare Part B helps to pay for covered services provided by a doctor, whether it be in his or her office, in the patient's home, or in a skilled-nursing facility. The major doctors' services covered are medical and surgical services, including the following:

Anesthesia

Diagnostic tests and procedures that are part of the patient's treatment

X rays and other radiology and pathology services

Nursing services

Drugs and biologicals that cannot be self-administered

Transfusions

Supplies

Physical and occupational therapy

Speech therapy

Services *not* covered include the following:

Routine physical examinations and tests related to routine examinations received as an outpatient

Routine foot care

Routine eye or hearing examinations

Immunizations (except pneumococcal vaccinations or immunizations required because of an injury or immediate risk of infection, and hepatitis B for certain persons at risk)

Cosmetic surgery (unless it is needed because of an accidental injury or to improve the function of a malformed part of the body)

Second Surgical Opinions

Medicare will cover all of the costs of a second surgical opinion for elective surgery. If the second opinion does not agree with the first Medicare will also cover the cost of the third opinion. Medicare operates a second-opinion referral center for the names and phone numbers of local doctors who will provide second opinions. State Peer Review Organizations (PROs) are responsible for reviewing the services provided by hospitals. Depending on state guidelines, PROs may require second opinions for some surgeries.

Chiropractor Services

The only chiropractic service that Medicare helps to pay for is the manual manipulation of the spine to correct a specific problem that can be demonstrated by X ray. Medicare will not cover the cost of the X ray. Beneficiaries who need X rays should have them taken by a physician rather than the chiropractor. Medicare will not pay for the diagnostic or therapeutic services of a chiropractor.

Podiatrist Services

Medicare will help pay for many services of a podiatrist except for routine foot care, treatment for flat feet or other structural misalignments, and removal of corns, calluses, and most warts. Medicare does make an exception for those with medical conditions such as diabetes that affect the lower limbs.

Dental Care

Medicare will only help pay for dental care if it involves surgery of the jaw or related structures, setting fractures, or services that would be covered if provided by a doctor. Routine dental care is not covered.

Optometrist Services

Medicare will help pay for the vision-care services of optometrists if the services are among those already covered by Medicare and if the optometrist is legally authorized to perform such services in the state he or she practices in.

Home Health Care

Under Part B, Medicare will also pay for the home health care that is described in Chapter 2.

Outpatient Hospital Services

Part B will help pay for emergency or outpatient services, tests, X rays and other radiology services, supplies, drugs and biologicals, and blood.

Mental-Health Services

Medicare will help pay for mental-health care for treatment of mental illness as long as a doctor certifies that the treatment is necessary and that without treatment the patient would require hospitalization. Medicare pays 50 percent of approved charges for services from comprehensive outpatient rehabilitation facilities, doctors, physician assistants, and psychologists and 80 percent for hospital outpatient treatment.

Ambulatory Surgical Services

Medicare will help pay for covered services in a Medicare-certified ambulatory surgical center. Such services can include pre- and postoperative care.

Outpatient Physical and Occupational Therapy and Speech Pathology Services

Medicare Part B will help pay for medically necessary outpatient physical and occupational therapy or speech pathology services when the following conditions are met:

The service is prescribed by a doctor

The doctor or therapist sets up a plan of treatment

The doctor periodically reviews the plan

Comprehensive Outpatient Rehabilitation Facility Services

Under limited circumstances Medicare will help pay for outpatient services in a comprehensive outpatient rehabilitation facility (CORF). Covered services include physician services, physical speech, occupational and respiratory therapies, counseling, and other related services.

Independent Clinical Laboratory Services

Part B pays the full approved fee for several covered clinical diagnostic tests provided by laboratories that are certified to perform them. The laboratory may not bill the beneficiary for the tests. A doctor who furnishes clinical diagnostic tests must accept assignment for such services. He or she may not bill the patient for them.

Portable Diagnostic X-Ray Services

Part B will pay the approved charge for portable diagnostic X-ray services received in the home if they are ordered by a doctor and if they are provided by a Medicare-certified supplier.

Ambulance Transportation

Part B will pay for medically necessary ambulance transportation if the ambulance, equipment, and personnel meet Medicare requirements and transportation in any other vehicle would endanger the patient's health. Medicare will not pay for ambulance transportation from an individual's home to the doctor's office. It will also only pay for transportation to the nearest hospital, even if the beneficiary's physician does not treat patients there.

Durable Medical Equipment

Medicare will help pay for equipment such as oxygen equipment and wheelchairs that a doctor prescribes for use in the home. In general, such equipment that costs more than $150 must be rented. If the beneficiary purchases used equipment, Medicare will waive the 20 percent coinsurance under certain circumstances. Beneficiaries should not take the word of the company selling or renting the equipment that Medicare will reimburse for it, but should check with a physician first.

Blood

Medicare will help pay for blood and blood components. However, the first three pints used in a calendar year must be replaced, or a replacement fee must be paid.

Prosthetic Devices

Medicare can help pay for devices needed to substitute for an internal body organ such as lenses needed after a cataract operation, colostomy or ileostomy bags, breast prostheses after a mastectomy, artificial limbs and eyes, and arm, leg, and neck braces.

Orthopedic shoes are covered only when they are part of leg braces and the cost is included in the orthopedist's charge. Dental plates and other orthodontal devices are not covered.

Medical Supplies

Part B can also help pay for supplies ordered by a doctor in connection with medical treatment such as surgical dressings, splints, and casts. Common first-aid supplies are not covered.

Other Covered Services

Part B can also help pay for rural health services; dialysis; physician's assistant, certified registered-nurse anesthetist, nurse-midwife, and psychological services; and for antigens and blood-clotting factors.

THINGS TO REMEMBER

As previously mentioned, beneficiaries should be sure that they know what services are covered under Medicare. Never assume that a service is or is not covered. For example, many Medicare recipients assume that routine office visits to physicians are covered; they are not. On the other hand, many assume that Medicare never pays for eyeglasses. But Medicare always pays for eyeglasses, including the frames, after a beneficiary has had cataract surgery.

Most important, it is always worthwhile for Medicare beneficiaries to select and use providers who accept assignment, which is often referred to as "participating." Details of selecting doctors and other health providers who accept assignment follow in the next chapter.

Chapter 4

Paying for
Medicare Coverage
and Collecting Benefits

MEDICARE COSTS AND REIMBURSEMENT FACTS

- The monthly Medicare Part B premium has increased from $17.90 in 1987 to $28.60 in 1990.

- As of 1990 the Part B deductible has remained stable at $75 for a number of years.

- Medicare medical-insurance payments are based on what the law defines as reasonable charges that are approved by the Medicare carrier in each area. Medicare will not make payment on charges that have not been approved.

- Using the "assignment method" for Part B services can save valuable health-care dollars. Participating physicians and suppliers are listed in state directories published by the state's Medicare carrier.

- Most Part A facilities will submit their bills to Medicare, and there is no need for the beneficiary to do anything.

- Beneficiaries no longer have to submit claims to Medicare for Part B services. *The doctor or other provider submits claims directly to the Medicare carrier.* However, claims for procedures prior to September 1, 1990, must be submitted to Medicare using form 1490S.

- After a claim has been processed, beneficiaries receive a written notice describing Medicare's decision on both Medicare Part A and Part B claims.

Introduction

This chapter covers the costs that Medicare recipients have as beneficiaries, the saving of health-care dollars through use of the Part B assignment method, the procedure for getting reimbursed for services, and the way approved charges for health services are determined.

Part B Costs

From the older health consumer's point of view, Part B is the most expensive and complicated part of the Medicare program. There is no charge for Part A, Medicare's hospital insurance, although it does require copayments and deductibles, which are detailed in Chapter 1. Part B of Medicare's payment structure is based on the concept of cost-sharing. *It pays a portion of the costs of medical care.* Beneficiaries pay a monthly premium, an annual deductible, a coinsurance amount, and any excess charges from a physician or other supplier. (For information on excess charges for nonassigned claims, see page 46.) The following provides details on Medicare Part B monthly premiums, the annual deductible, and the coinsurance.

Part B Monthly Premiums

Beneficiaries must pay monthly premiums, which rise annually. Increases in the premium have been the cause of a great deal of concern recently. Most beneficiaries elect to have premiums deducted from their monthly Social Security checks. Otherwise they are billed quarterly.

Part B Annual Deductibles

The Part B annual deductible consists of a specified amount of Part B "approved charges." As of 1990 the deductible has remained stable at $75 for a number of years. The deductible must be paid before Medicare will reimburse the beneficiary or provider for any services. Medicare will notify beneficiaries as to whether they have met their deductible or not.

Part B Coinsurance

As previously mentioned, Part B was designed to pay 80 percent of the cost of covered services, after payment of the deductible. Beneficiaries pay the other 20 percent, which is called the Part B coinsurance, as well as any excess charges above Medicare's approved amount. A few services such as home health benefits and second opinions for surgery are exempt from coinsurance.

Unless the provider accepts assignment, Medicare beneficiaries often wind up paying more than 20 percent. (See page 46 for information on assignment.) Fees charged by doctors and other suppliers of Part B services vary, even within one area. *But Medicare has a fixed schedule of fees, called the approved amount, for procedures done in specific areas. Medicare will pay only 80 percent of that approved amount.* If bills from doctors and other Part B suppliers are higher than the approved amount, the beneficiary must pay the difference.

Purchasing Medicare Coverage

Persons age 65 and older who don't qualify for Medicare may purchase coverage. (See Figure 1.2.) The individual must have been a citizen or permanent resident alien for the past five years. Enrollment is limited to the period between January 1 and March 31 each year. (This is often referred to as an open-enrollment period.) Coverage begins July 1 of the year of enrollment.

For both programs, it is most economical to enroll within the period three months before turning 65, during the birthday month, or four months after the sixty-fifth birthday. Individuals who are working and over age 65 with employer health plans can wait to enroll in Part B until the special enrollment period during the year of their retirement (see below). They won't have to pay the 10 percent premium surcharge if they meet certain requirements.

Enrolling in Part B When Eligible for Part A

Beneficiaries who are receiving Medicare Part A but elected at some point *not* to receive Part B may change their minds and enroll for medical insurance, using HCFA Form 40B (Figure 4.1), during Medicare's open-enrollment season between January 1 and March 31 each year.

The premiums for both Part A and Part B are costly. For Part A, if the individual enrolls during an open-enrollment period that begins more than one year after his or her sixty-fifth birthday, *the monthly premium is 10 percent higher than what Medicare calls the basic premium amount, which is the base used for determining the monthly charge.* (The basic premium amount for 1990 is $175 a month.) For Part B, if the older individual enrolls during a general-enrollment period, *the monthly premium is 10 percent higher than the basic premium for each 12-month period during which he or she could have had medical insurance but did not enroll.* The basic medical-insurance premium was $27.90 a month through December 31, 1989.

Using the Assignment Method for Part B Services

Using the assignment method for Part B services can save valuable health-care dollars. The assignment method involves using Part B providers who offer their patients a more economical alternative than those who "balance bill" (see below). They do this by participating in Medicare's program for minimizing patients' out-of-pocket costs. Participants in the program agree to "accept assignment," meaning that they agree to accept Medicare's approved or allowed charge *as payment in full. They will not charge the beneficiary more than the 20 percent of Medicare's rate that he or she must always pay as a share of Part B costs.*

APPLICATION FOR ENROLLMENT IN MEDICARE
THE MEDICAL INSURANCE PROGRAM

TID ENR

1. SOCIAL SECURITY CLAIM NUMBER

2. FOR AGENCY USE ONLY

(CAN) □ □ □ - □ □ - □ □ □ □

(BIC)

3. DO YOU WISH TO ENROLL FOR MEDICAL INSURANCE UNDER MEDICARE?

(DEC)   YES □   NO □

4. YOUR NAME

(CLN)   FIRST   MIDDLE INITIAL   SURNAME

5. PRINT SOCIAL SECURITY NUMBER HOLDER'S NAME IF DIFFERENT FROM YOURS

6. MAILING ADDRESS (NUMBER AND STREET, P.O. BOX, OR ROUTE)

IF THIS IS A CHANGE OF ADDRESS, CHECK HERE □

7. CITY, STATE, AND ZIP CODE

8. TELEPHONE NUMBER

9. WRITTEN SIGNATURE (DO NOT PRINT)

10. DATE SIGNED

SIGN HERE ⟶ _____

11. IF THIS APPLICATION HAS BEEN SIGNED BY MARK (X), A WITNESS WHO KNOWS THE
APPLICANT MUST SUPPLY THE INFORMATION REQUESTED BELOW

12. SIGNATURE OF WITNESS

13. DATE SIGNED

14. ADDRESS OF WITNESS

15. REMARKS

FORM HCFA — 40 B (8-82)

Figure 4.1   Application for Medical Insurance under Medicare. Form HCFA-40B.

Figure 4.1   (continued)

SPECIAL MESSAGE FOR INDIVIDUAL APPLYING
FOR MEDICAL INSURANCE UNDER MEDICARE

This form is your application for the medical insurance part of Medicare. It can be used either during your personal enrollment period or during any general enrollment period.

Your personal enrollment period lasts for 7 months. It begins 3 months before the month you reach age 65 (or 3 months before the 25th month you have received social security disability benefits) and it ends 3 months after you reach age 65 (or 3 months after the 25th month you have received social security disability benefits). To have medical insurance start in the month you are 65 (or the 25th month of disability insurance benefits), you must sign up in the first 3 months of your personal enrollment period. If you sign up in any of the remaining 4 months, your medical insurance starting date will be later.

If you do not file during your personal enrollment period, you can file any time after that during a general enrollment period which is the first 3 months of every year. If you sign up in a general enrollment period, your medical insurance begins July 1 of that year. However, when you file in a general enrollment period, your premium may be subject to a penalty increase. For each 12 month period elapsing between the end of your personal enrollment period and the general enrollment period in which you file, your premium will be increased 10 percent.

Physicians and other providers who do not accept assignment "balance bill" or "charge for the excess," which means that they bill patients for costs above Medicare's approved or allowed charge. Physicians and other providers who do not accept assignment and "balance bill" are not necessarily better. In this case cost is not in itself an indication of higher quality.

Assignment rates have increased dramatically over the past several years. According to an analysis by the U.S. Congress Committee on Ways and Means, 80 percent of covered Medicare charges are now assigned. However, according to the Physician Payment Review Commission, only half of all Medicare beneficiaries and 38 percent of poor beneficiaries know about the program.

The following two examples and Table 4.1 illustrate the benefits of using the assignment method.

Mrs. Smith's doctor does not accept assignment and charges her $100 for a medical procedure, but Medicare's approved charge is only $60. Medicare will pay 80 percent of $60, which is $48. Medicare then will have met its obligation. Mrs. Smith will have to pay the 20 percent: $12. However, she will also have to make up the difference between the $100 bill and Medicare's $60 approved amount. This is the *excess charge* or *balance billing,* which in Mrs. Smith's case is $40. Her total bill is $52.

Mr. Jones goes to a doctor who accepts assignment. Mr. Jones pays 20 percent of Medicare's approved charge of $60, or $12, for the procedure Mrs. Smith paid $52 for.

Fortunately for Medicare consumers, physicians and providers can sign an annual contract with Medicare agreeing to always accept assignment for Medicare patients. These providers are said to be "participating." Other doctors may accept assignment some of the time, while others may not accept it at all. Medicare beneficiaries should find out, before treatment, whether their doctor or other Part B supplier accepts assignment.

Table 4.1   Saving Money through Assignment: A Comparison of Two Claims for the Same Procedure

	MRS. SMITH'S BILL (not assigned)	MR. JONES' BILL (assigned)
Doctor's Charge	$100	$60
Medicare's Approved Amount	$60	$60
Difference (doctor's excess charge)	$40	$0
Amount Medicare Pays	$48 (80% of $60)	$48 (80% of $60)
Amount Patient Pays	$52 (20% of $60 + doctor's excess charge of $40–$52)	$12 (20% of $60)

Here is a quick review of the assignment method:

The assignment method can save valuable health-care dollars.

Using the assignment method means selecting providers who agree to accept Medicare's approved charge as total payment.

The beneficiary then pays no more than the annual deductible and 20 percent of the approved charge.

Some providers of Part B services submit claims for patients but do not accept assignment. Beneficiaries should make sure that any provider agreeing to submit claims to Medicare also accepts assignment.

Locating Physicians and Suppliers Who Accept Assignment

Participating physicians and suppliers are listed in state directories published by the state's Medicare carrier. Copies of the publication, the *Medicare-Participating Physician/Supplier Directory*, or *Medpard*, may be purchased from state Medicare carriers (listed in Part Two) or reviewed in a Social Security, Railroad Retirement, or Area Agency on Aging office. Beneficiaries should look for a Medicare participating sign in the office of a particular physician or other provider. In addition, seniors can ask individual physicians or suppliers whether they "participate," which means they have agreed to accept assignment for all

```
┌────────────────────────────────────────────────────────────────┐
│                  MEDICARE  BENEFIT  NOTICE                       │
│                                          DATE                    │
│   BENEFICIARY  NAME  AND  ADDRESS        MEDICARE  NUMBER        │
│                                                                  │
│   SERVICES  FURNISHED  BY    DATE(S)     BENEFITS  USED          │
│   ─────────────────────────────────────────────────────────     │
│   UNIVERSITY  HOSPITAL       X/XX/XX     04  INPATIENT  HOSPITAL  DAY │
│                              THRU                                 │
│                              X/XX/XX                             │
│                                                                  │
│   PAYMENT  STATUS                                                │
│   ─────────────────────────────────────────────────────────     │
│   MEDICARE  PAID  ALL  COVERED  SERVICES  EXCEPT:                │
│   $560  FOR  THE  INPATIENT  DEDUCTIBLE                          │
│   ─────────────────────────────────────────────────────────     │
│                                                                  │
│                                                                  │
│                                                                  │
│                                                                  │
└────────────────────────────────────────────────────────────────┘
```

This notice provides information on the amount of money Medicare is paying for a specified Part A claim. It is NOT a bill.

Figure 4.2   Sample of a Medicare Benefit Notice.

Medicare patients. Even if the answer is no, many will make an exception and will say yes on special request.

Many geriatric clinics accept assignment for all patients, which means that they are a "participating" geriatric clinic. Most provide additional complementary services such as case management and counseling. Geriatric clinics are not listed in the *Medpard*; generally they locate patients through advertising.

Collecting Payment from Medicare

Most Part A facilities will submit their bills to Medicare, and there is no need for the beneficiary to do anything. Medicare pays benefits directly to the hospital or other facility. Whenever a facility sends Medicare a bill for payment, Medicare in turn sends the beneficiary a Medicare Benefit Notice explaining the decision made on the claim. Sometimes these notices are confusing, and recipients think they are bills. Beneficiaries with questions should contact the office shown on the notice. (See Figure 4.2.)

Medicare's process for paying its share of Part B costs has been greatly streamlined to the advantage of the beneficiary. For all Part B services after September 1, 1990, *the doctor or other provider submits claims for the beneficiary. The beneficiary does not have to send a form or bill to the Medicare carrier.* However, for services received before September 1, 1990, if the provider does not accept assignment or does not submit a claim as a special service for patients, the beneficiary *will* have to submit claims to the Medicare carrier. Claims must be submitted using Form 1490S, "Request for Medical Payment." Forms are available at doctors', Social Security, or Medicare carriers' offices.

Basically, beneficiaries have 15 months to submit claims. A good rule to follow is to submit claims as soon as possible. Supplemental insurance companies, which require information on how much Medicare has paid before they will process a claim, also have time limits on when claims can be submitted. If the claim was made to Medicare too late and there was a delay in processing it, there may not be time to process the supplemental-coverage claim.

On the back of the claim form are instructions on how to fill out the form. The form has to be filled out accurately to avoid delay in payment. An itemized bill must be submitted with the claim. It must show:

The date the service was received

The place where the service was received

A description of the service and codes

The charge for each service

The doctor or supplier who provided the service

The beneficiary's name and Social Security number, including the letter at the end of the number

If the bill does not include all this information, payment will be delayed. It is also helpful if the nature of the illness is shown on the bill. Senior-health-insurance counselors recommend that beneficiaries submit a separate claim for each provider. Otherwise the beneficiary will receive one check for a number of providers, and it will be up to him or her to figure out what portion of the bill goes to what provider.

Regardless of who submits the claim to Medicare, before any medical-insurance payment is made, the record must show that the beneficiary has met the deductible ($75 in 1990). If the bills amount to less than $75, Medicare will not reimburse any portion

FORM APPROVED
OMB NO. 0938-0008

PATIENT'S REQUEST FOR MEDICAL PAYMENT

IMPORTANT—SEE OTHER SIDE FOR INSTRUCTIONS

PLEASE TYPE OR PRINT INFORMATION   MEDICAL INSURANCE BENEFITS SOCIAL SECURITY ACT

NOTICE: Anyone who misrepresents or falsifies essential information requested by this form may upon conviction be subject to fine and imprisonment under Federal Law. No Part B Medicare benefits may be paid unless this form is received as required by existing law and regulations (20 CFR 422.510).

1 Name of Beneficiary from Health Insurance Card
(First)   (Middle)   (Last)

SEND COMPLETED FORM TO:

2 Claim Number from Health Insurance Card

Patient's Sex
☐ Male
☐ Female

3 Patient's Mailing Address (City, State, Zip Code)
Check here if this is a new address ——————— ☐

(Street or P.O. Box — Include Apartment Number)

(City)   (State)   (Zip)

3b Telephone Number
(Include Area Code)

(___ ___ ___)

___ ___ ___ — ___ ___ ___ ___

4 Describe the Illness or Injury for which Patient Received Treatment

4b Was condition related to:
A. Patient's employment
☐ Yes   ☐ No

B. Accident
☐ Auto   ☐ Other

4c Was patient being treated with chronic dialysis or kidney transplant?
☐ Yes   ☐ No

5 a. Are you employed and covered under an employee health plan?
☐ Yes   ☐ No

b. Is your spouse employed and are you covered under your spouse's employee health plan?
☐ Yes   ☐ No

c. If you have any medical coverage other than Medicare, such as private insurance, employment related insurance, State Agency (Medicaid), or the VA, complete:
Name and Address of other insurance, State Agency (Medicaid), or VA office

Policy or Medical Assistance No.

Policyholders Name:

NOTE: If you DO NOT want payment information on this claim released, put an (X) here ——————— ☐

6 I AUTHORIZE ANY HOLDER OF MEDICAL OR OTHER INFORMATION ABOUT ME TO RELEASE TO THE SOCIAL SECURITY ADMINISTRATION AND HEALTH CARE FINANCING ADMINISTRATION OR ITS INTERMEDIARIES OR CARRIERS ANY INFORMATION NEEDED FOR THIS OR A RELATED MEDICARE CLAIM. I PERMIT A COPY OF THIS AUTHORIZATION TO BE USED IN PLACE OF THE ORIGINAL, AND REQUEST PAYMENT OF MEDICAL INSURANCE BENEFITS TO ME.

Signature of Patient (If patient is unable to sign, see Block 6 on reverse)

6b Date signed

IMPORTANT
ATTACH ITEMIZED BILLS FROM YOUR DOCTOR(S) OR SUPPLIER(S) TO THE BACK OF THIS FORM

FORM HCFA-1490S (7-85)   DEPARTMENT OF HEALTH AND HUMAN SERVICES—HEALTH CARE FINANCING ADMINISTRATION

Figure 4.3   Request for Medical Payment. Form HCFA-1490S.

Figure 4.3 (continued)

HOW TO FILL OUT THIS MEDICARE FORM

Medicare will pay you directly when you complete this form and attach an itemized bill from your doctor or supplier. Your bill does not have to be paid before you submit this claim for payment, but you MUST attach an itemized bill in order for Medicare to process this claim.

FOLLOW THESE INSTRUCTIONS CAREFULLY:

A. Completion of this form.

Block 1.	Print your name **exactly** as it is shown on your Medicare Card.
Block 2.	Print your Health Insurance Claim Number including the letter at the end **exactly** as it is shown on your Medicare card. Check the appropriate box for the patient's sex.
Block 3.	Furnish your mailing address and include your telephone number in Block 3b.
Block 4.	Describe the illness or injury for which you received treatment. Check the appropriate box in Blocks 4b and 4c.
Block 5a.	Complete this Block if you are between the ages of 65 and 69 and enrolled in a health insurance plan where you are currently working.
Block 5b.	Complete this Block if you are between the ages of 65 and 69 and enrolled in a health insurance plan where your spouse is currently working.
Block 5c.	Complete this Block if you have any medical coverage other than Medicare. Be sure to provide the Policy or Medical Assistance Number. You may check the box provided if you do not wish payment information from this claim released to your other insurer.
Block 6.	Be sure to sign your name. If you cannot write your name, make an (X) mark. Then have a witness sign his or her name and address in Block 6 too.
	If you are completing this form for another Medicare patient you should write (By) and sign your name and address in Block 6. You also should show your relationship to the patient and briefly explain why the patient cannot sign.
Block 6b.	Print the date you completed this form.

B. Each itemized bill MUST show all of the following information:

*   Date of each service

*   Place of each service —Doctor's Office —Independent Laboratory
                            —Outpatient Hospital —Nursing Home
                            —Patient's Home —Inpatient Hospital

*   Description of each surgical or medical service or supply furnished.

*   Charge for EACH service.

*   Doctor's or supplier's name and address. Many times a bill will show the names of several doctors or suppliers. IT IS VERY IMPORTANT THE ONE WHO TREATED YOU BE IDENTIFIED. Simply circle his/her name on the bill.

*   It is helpful if the diagnosis is shown on the physician's bill. If not, be sure you have completed Block 4 of this form.

*   Mark out any services on the bill(s) you are attaching for which you have already filed a Medicare claim.

*   If the patient is deceased please contact your Social Security office for instructions on how to file a claim.

*   Attach an Explanation of Medicare Benefits notice from the other insurer if you are also requesting Medicare payment.

COLLECTION AND USE OF MEDICARE INFORMATION

We are authorized by the Health Care Financing Administration to ask you for information needed in the administration of the Medicare program. Authority to collect information is in section 205 (a), 1872 and 1875 of the Social Security Act, as amended.

The information we obtain to complete your Medicare claim is used to identify you and to determine your eligibility. It is also used to decide if the services and supplies you received are covered by Medicare and to insure that proper payment is made.

The information may also be given to other providers of services, carriers, intermediaries, medical review boards, and other organizations as necessary to administer the Medicare program. For example, it may be necessary to disclose information about the Medicare benefits you have used to a hospital or doctor.

With one exception, which is discussed below, there are no penalties under social security law for refusing to supply information. However, failure to furnish information regarding the medical services rendered or the amount charged would prevent payment of the claim. Failure to furnish any other information, such as name or claim number, would delay payment of the claim.

It is mandatory that you tell us if you are being treated for a work related injury so we can determine whether worker's compensation will pay for the treatment. Section 1877 (a) (3) of the Social Security Act provides criminal penalties for withholding this information.

☆U.S. Government Printing Office: 1986—608-697

of the bill. The Health Care Financing Administration recommends that once a beneficiary has collected enough bills to meet the deductible, he or she immediately send Form 1490S to the appropriate carrier (listed in Part Two).

Beneficiaries should keep the following for their own records:

Copies of the claim form and any bills submitted

Records of the deductible for each year

The Medicare Medical Insurance Claims Record (Figure 4.4) can be used for keeping track of Part B claims. Social Security used to supply beneficiaries with the form, but it is now out of print. It can, however, be copied for personal use or distribution. Schedules for submitting Part B claims follow.

For Service between the Following Dates	A Claim Must Be Submitted By
Oct. 1, 1988–Sept. 30, 1989	Dec. 31, 1990
Oct. 1, 1989–Sept. 30, 1990	Dec. 30, 1991
Oct. 1, 1990–Sept. 30, 1990	Dec. 31, 1992

Medicare payments are handled by private insurance organizations under contract with the government. Intermediaries handle claims from hospitals, skilled-nursing facilities, and home health agencies. Carriers handle claims under Part B. These are usually private insurance companies that have contracts with Medicare to handle the details of processing and paying claims. Claims are to be filed in the state where the service or treatment was performed. (Carrier addresses are listed in Part Two.)

There are special rules for submitting claims for beneficiaries who are members of health maintenance organizations (HMOs). Medicare HMO members who receive bills for health services should consult their HMO handbooks.

It is worth reviewing the following important fact about Medicare reimbursement: *Medicare beneficiaries should be sure that any health-service provider they use is approved for Medicare payments.* Medicare will not pay for care received from nonparticipating (not Medicare-approved) hospitals, skilled-

Medicare Medical Insurance Claims Record

Note: You can use the "Other Remarks" column to keep track of your medical insurance deductible until it's met or for notes about appeals or private supplementary insurance.

Date you mailed claim	Date of service or supply	Doctor or supplier who provided service or supply	Service or supply you received	Charge for service or supply	Date and amount of Medicare payment	Other Remarks

Form SSA-3596 (12-79)
Prior editions may be used until supply is exhausted

GPO : 1980 O - 309-960

Figure 4.4   Medicare Medical Insurance Claims Record. Form SSA-3596.

nursing facilities, home health agencies, or hospices. There is one exception—Medicare will pay if the individual has been sent to a nonparticipating hospital in an emergency and if the hospital is the closest one equipped to handle the problem.

Notice of Payment by Medicare

After a claim has been processed, beneficiaries will receive a written notice that describes Medicare's decision on both Medicare Part A and Part B claims. (See Table 4.2.) With a few exceptions, notices are sent out regardless of whether the beneficiary or health-care provider submitted the bill for reimbursement. Sometimes these notices are confusing, and recipients think they are bills. Beneficiaries with questions should contact the office shown on the notice.

The notice for an inpatient hospital or skilled-nursing stay is called a "Medicare Benefit Notice." (See Figure 4.2.) A "Medicare Claims Information" notice (see Figure 4.5) is sent to beneficiaries for Part B services received through Part A facilities. For example, a patient who went to a hospital outpatient facility for radiation treatments would receive a "Medicare Claims Information" notice rather than a "Medicare Benefit Notice." This is a record of Part B benefits used. The notice of Medicare's decision for home health services is usually described in a letter indicating either payment or denial. With the exception of outpatient hospital services, all other Part B services are included in "Explanation of Medicare Benefits," often referred to by its initials, EOMB. (See Figure 4.6.)

In addition, Medicare automatically sends some claims to private supplemental insurance companies through an agreement

Table 4.2   Medicare Claims Processing

	PART A	PART B
Claims Processing	Intermediaries	Carriers
Who Submits the Bill	Providers	Providers, after Sept. 1, 1990
Notice Received	Medicare Benefits Notice	Explanation of Medicare Benefits (EOMB) or Medicare Claims Information for Part B Services Received or a Letter from the Provider

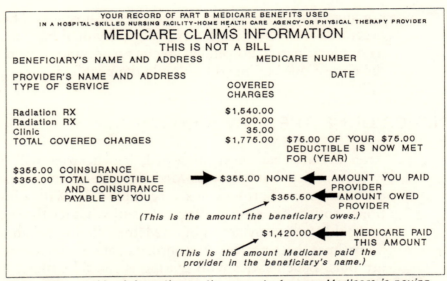

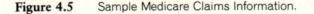

This notice provides information on the amount of money Medicare is paying for a specified Part B service received through a Part A provider. It is NOT a bill.

Figure 4.5   Sample Medicare Claims Information.

with Medicare, saving paperwork for the beneficiary. Beneficiaries should check with their supplemental insurance companies to see whether this service is available.

When a Relative Dies

When a beneficiary dies, problems arise for Part B claims for providers who do not accept assignment. (Medicare will pay all other claims directly to Part A providers and to Part B providers who accept assignment.)

Medicare encourages a representative who is willing to take responsibility for the deceased's bills to sign a "Request for Information—Medicare Payment for Services to a Patient Now Deceased." (See Figure 4.7.) *No one, including a spouse, is obligated to sign this form. If they do, they agree to be responsible for paying the provider in full.* (See Chapter 8.) Medicare then sends the money directly to the signer of the form.

```
┌─────────────────────────────────────────────────────────────────┐
│              YOUR EXPLANATION OF MEDICARE BENEFITS                │
│       READ THIS NOTICE CAREFULLY AND KEEP IT FOR YOUR RECORDS     │
│                      THIS IS NOT A BILL                          │
│                                                                   │
│  HEALTH CARE FINANCING ADMINISTRATION          DATE              │
│  BENEFICIARY'S NAME AND ADDRESS          CARRIER'S NAME AND ADDRESS│
│                                                                   │
│  ASSIGNMENT WAS NOT TAKEN ON YOUR CLAIM FOR $485.50              │
│  (This message explains if assignment was taken on the           │
│  claim.)                                                          │
│                                                 BILLED   APPROVED │
│                                                 $485.00  $250.50  │
│  A.E. SMITH        ANESTHESIA      DATE                           │
│  (This message explains what the bill is for and gives the       │
│  billed vs. approved amount.)                                    │
│                                                                   │
│  TOTAL APPROVED AMOUNT                                  $250.50  │
│  MEDICARE PAYMENT (20% OF THE APPROVED AMOUNT)          $200.40  │
│  (This message explains how much Medicare is paying              │
│  toward the approved charge.)                                    │
│                                                                   │
│  WE ARE PAYING A TOTAL OF $200.40 TO YOU ON THE ENCLOSED         │
│  CHECK. PLEASE CASH IT AS SOON AS POSSIBLE. IF YOU HAVE          │
│  OTHER INSURANCE IT MAY HELP YOU WITH THE PART MEDICARE DOES     │
│  NOT PAY.                                                        │
│                                                                   │
│          (YOU HAVE MET THE DEDUCTIBLE FOR 1989)                 │
│  (This message explains how much of the Part B deductible       │
│  has been met for the calendar year.)                           │
└─────────────────────────────────────────────────────────────────┘
```

This notice provides information on the amount of money Medicare is paying for a specified Part B claim. It is NOT a bill.

Figure 4.6   Sample Explanation of Medicare Benefits (EOMB).

How Approved Charges Are Determined

Medicare medical-insurance payments are based on what the law defines as reasonable charges that are approved by the Medicare carrier in each area. *Medicare will not make payment on charges that have not been approved.* Each year the carrier for a particular area reviews the actual charges made by doctors and suppliers in the area during the previous year. These actual charges are then compared to what are called the customary charge (the median charge for that provider) and the prevailing charge (the amount that will cover three out of four customary charges in a geographic area) for that service. Based on this review, new charges are put into effect about October 1 of each year. This method is controversial, and many providers assert that the new figures are based on outdated information, causing unreasonably low reimbursement rates.

60

DEPARTMENT OF HEALTH AND HUMAN SERVICES
HEALTH CARE FINANCING ADMINISTRATION

Form Approved
OMB No. 0938-0020

REQUEST FOR INFORMATION — MEDICARE PAYMENT FOR SERVICES TO A PATIENT NOW DECEASED

No further monies or other benefits may be paid out under this program unless this report is completed and filed as required by existing law and regulations (20 C.F.R. 405 1683).

When completed, send this form to:	Deceased patient
	Health insurance claim number of deceased patient

For Services Provided By:

PART I — PAID BILL (If The Bill Is Not Paid Go To Part II)

If bills for medical or other health services were paid by or for the deceased person, Medicare benefits may be due. We hope you will be able to help us determine who should receive payment. The person who paid the deceased's bill(s) has first right to any payment due. If the deceased or his estate paid the bill(s), benefits will be paid to the legal representative of the estate. If there is no legal representative, payment will be made to the person who stands highest in the list of relatives below. If the person who paid the bill(s) dies before being reimbursed, payment is also made to the person standing highest in the list of relatives. If there are no living relatives or legal representatives, no payment will be made. Please answer the questions, sign on the reverse side and return this form in the enclosed envelope.

ALWAYS INCLUDE EVIDENCE OF PAYMENT SUCH AS A RECEIPTED BILL OR OTHER RECEIPT

1. Who paid the deceased's bills for medical or other health services?

☐ The deceased or his estate *(Answer (2) below)*

☐ Yourself *(Sign on reverse side and return form)*

☐ Other person or organization (Enter the person's or organization's name and address in item 4 below. If there is more than one person or organization, attach a listing of names and addresses of these persons or organizations to this form.

2. Is there a legal representative of the estate?

☐ Yes *(If "Yes," print his name and address below, Sign on reverse side and return form)*. If you are the legal representative, submit a copy of your appointment papers with this form.

☐ No *(If "No," answer item 3 below.*

3. This item is aswered only if item 2 above is checked "No". Put a check in the box next to the living relative that stands highest on the following list and then write that relative's name and address in item 4 below. (If you check the box for child or children and there is more than one child, attach a listing of the names and address of all the children to this form.)

☐ Widow or widower living in the same household as the deceased at the time of death, or entitled to a monthly Social Security or Railroad Retirement benefit on the same earnings record as the deceased in the month of death.

☐ A child or children of the deceased entitled to monthly Social Security or Railroad Retirement benefits or the same earnings record as the deceased in the month of death. *(List the names and addresses of all entitled children of the deceased)*

☐ A parent or parents of the deceased entitled to monthly Social Security or Railroad Retirement benefits on the same earnings record as the deceased in the month of death.

☐ A widow or widower who was neither living with the deceased at the time of death nor at that time entitled on the same earnings record to a Social Security or Railroad Retirement benefit.

☐ A child or children of the deceased who were not entitled in the month of death to monthly Social Security or Railroad Retirement benefits on the same earnings record as the deceased. *(List the names and addresses of all such children.)*

☐ A parent or parents not entitled in the month of death to monthly Social Security or Railroad Retirement benefits on the same earnings record as the deceased.

4. Name	Address

FORM HCFA-1660 (8-81)   DESTROY PRIOR EDITIONS

Continued On Back

Figure 4.7   Request for Information. Form HCFA-1660.

Figure 4.7   (continued)

PART II — UNPAID BILL (If The Bill Is Paid, Complete Part I)

When the beneficiary has died and a physician or supplier does not agree to accept the reasonable charge as the full charge, payment may be made on the basis of an unpaid bill to the person who has agreed to assume legal liability to pay the physician or supplier.

If you are assuming such legal liability and want to claim Medicare benefits for the services furnished to the deceased beneficiary, you must furnish the documents listed below to us and sign this form below. Your signature below certifies to the following statement:

I have assumed the legal obligation to pay the physician or supplier named below for services furnished to the deceased beneficiary on the date(s) indicated. I hereby claim any Medicare benefits due for these services.

Name of Physician or Supplier	Name of Deceased Beneficiary	Date(s) of Services

In addition furnish the following documents together with this form to us.

1. A completed form HCFA-1490S, PATIENT'S REQUEST FOR MEDICARE PAYMENTS. You must sign item 6 of the HCFA-1490S in lieu of the deceased beneficiary. (You may obtain a copy of the HCFA-1490S from a Social Security Office if you did not receive one with this form;) and

2. A signed statement from the physician or supplier which shows that the physician or supplier refuses to accept assignment for the bill; and

3. An itemized bill from the physician or supplier which identifies you as the person to whom the physician or supplier looks for payment.

Sign below and return this form together with the documents specified above to the address shown in the upper left portion of the form on the other side. If no carrier name and address is shown on the other side of this form request the proper addressee information from a Social Security Office.

I certify that if I receive the entire amount due, I will distribute it among other persons if they are legally entitled to it. Knowing that anyone making a false statement or representation of a material fact for use in determining the right to or the amount of Health Insurance benefits commits a crime punishable under the Federal law. I certify that the above statements are true.

If this statement has been signed by mark (X), two witnesses who know the claimant should sign below, giving their full addresses. The signature and title of a Social Security employee will suffice in lieu of signatures of two witnesses. Name	Name of claimant *(Please print)* Signature of claimant *(Write in ink)* **SIGN HERE** ▶
Address *(Number and Street, City, State and ZIP Code)*	Mailing Address *(Number and Street, P.O. Box or Route)*
Name	City, State and ZIP Code
Address *(Number and Street, City, State and ZIP Code)*	Date *(Month, Day and Year)* | Telephone number

If you wish assistance in completing this request, please take it to a Social Security Office. The people there will help you.
        PLEASE RETURN THIS REQUEST IN THE ENCLOSED ENVELOPE

HCFA-1660 (8-81)

When Medicare Is the Secondary Payer

There are times when Medicare is the secondary payer, which means that it pays after other insurance has paid first. This occurs at the following times:

When the beneficiary works after age 65 and is covered under an employer's group plan.

When the beneficiary is disabled (with an impairment other than kidney failure) and is covered under an employer's group plan.

When the beneficiary is in an accident and the automobile medical insurance or state no-fault insurance pays. The claim should be filed with Medicare after the other claims are filed first.

When the beneficiary is in an accident and liability insurance pays. In this case the claim should be filed with Medicare first. Medicare will get its payment back when liability insurance pays.

When the beneficiary is entitled to Medicare because of permanent kidney failure and is covered by an employer's health plan, Medicare will be the secondary payer during an initial period of up to 12 months. At the end of that period, Medicare becomes the primary payer.

Chapter 5

Beneficiaries' Rights To Appeal Medicare Claims

FACTS ON MEDICARE APPEALS

- As few as 3 percent of Medicare recipients appeal claims.

- Fifty percent of all appeals are won by beneficiaries.

- Medicare beneficiaries have ten important general areas of appeals rights under Medicare.

- When a problem arises it is important to act quickly to appeal a Medicare claim.

Introduction

When older adults have been denied benefits or feel that they are not receiving fair treatment under Medicare, they have the right to appeal for reconsideration to the agency in question or a higher court. In other words, they have the right to ask for a review of the case. Unfortunately, estimates of the number of Medicare beneficiaries who appeal are as low as 3 percent, although, ironically, about 50 percent of all appeals result in higher payments to beneficiaries.

There are two major reasons for the absence of Medicare appeals: a lack of beneficiary understanding of how Medicare works, and the fact that too often the very beneficiaries who have good reason to question Medicare's decisions on claims are also too ill to make appeals. However, many analysts believe that Medicare appeals will increase as a result of improved beneficiary education and a recent surge in senior-health-insurance counseling projects.

This chapter covers ten major areas of appeals rights under Medicare. Five of these rights fall under Medicare Part A, three fall under Medicare Part B, and two apply to both Part A and Part B. Many experts say that the most important of these appeals rights are early discharge from the hospital (1); denial of skilled-nursing-facility services, home health care, or hospice care (5); and claims for doctors' bills (6). The ten major appeals rights are the following:

Part A

1. Early discharge from the hospital (hospital notice of noncoverage for a continued stay)

2. Preadmission denial by a hospital

3. Hospital notice of noncoverage for admission that was not medically necessary

4. Notice of noncoverage as part of an automatic retrospective review by the peer review organization

5. Denial of skilled-nursing-facility services, home health services, or hospice care

Part B

6. Denial of a usually covered doctor's visit or other service

7. New information becomes available

8. Getting a lower Medicare payment than expected for a physician's service or other Part B claim

Parts A and B

9. Denial of eligibility for Medicare

10. Denial of "waiver of liability" in noncoverage situations

Who Can Appeal

As a general rule Part A appeals are initiated by the institution providing the service; in other words, the hospital, skilled nursing facility, home health agency, or hospice. Part B appeals can be initiated by beneficiaries, a representative of the beneficiary, or physicians or other Part B providers. In either case the most important rule is to act quickly to exert beneficiary rights.

Part A Appeals

Before setting a Part A appeal in motion, the provider in question must submit a claim to Medicare for services. *Otherwise the patient has no right to appeal.* Even if the nursing home or other Part A provider thinks that Medicare won't pay the claim and is reluctant to submit a bill to Medicare, *the beneficiary has the right to insist that a specific type of claim called a "no-payment billing" be submitted on his or her behalf.*

After the "no-payment billing" claim has been submitted, the provider and the individual will both receive a written copy of the decision from Medicare, called an "initial determination." The determination serves as the basis for instituting an appeal. The beneficiary has 60 days after receiving it to appeal.

The Medicare Part A appeal system has four important steps:

1. *The Reconsideration,* in which the beneficiary submits Form HCFA-2649 (see Figure 5.1) to the Peer Review Organization, intermediary, or carrier, asking that the case be reconsidered. The case is then reviewed based on the evidence and findings used in the first determination, and the beneficiary is informed of the decision in writing.

2. *The Social Security Administrative Hearing,* in which the beneficiary submits Form HA-5011 (see Figure 5.2) and an administrative law judge sets a time and location to examine evidence in person and to take testimony on the case. The beneficiary or a representative may appear. A hearing must be requested within six months.

3. *The Social Security Appeals Council Review,* in which the beneficiary submits Form HA-520 (see Figure 5.3) to the Appeals Council in Arlington, Virginia. The council may decide not to hear the case, may grant the request for a review and make a decision, or may send the case back to an administrative law judge for review. The Appeals Council Review is a paper review only. The beneficiary does not go before the council in person.

4. *The Civil Complaint to the Federal District Court,* in which the beneficiary makes a civil complaint to the Federal District Court. At this point it is usually best for the beneficiary to be represented by an attorney.

For steps 2 through 4 there are dollar minimums that the claim must meet.

Each of these steps can result in a decision that is favorable to the beneficiary. However, if the beneficiary is not satisfied with a decision at any stage in the appeals process and wants to continue, each individual step must be completed in order to go on to the next. In other words, a beneficiary who is not satisfied with the results of a Social Security Administrative Hearing (step 2) cannot decide to go to the Federal District Court next (step 4). He or she must try the Social Security Appeals Council first (step 3).

The following sections detail the reconsideration process, the initial step that beneficiaries must go through when appealing a case. Steps 2, 3, and 4 are basically the same for all types of Part A appeals. Peer Review Organizations (described below), fiscal intermediaries, and carriers will provide beneficiaries with details on how to follow the last three steps.

DRGs and Medicare's Prospective Payment System

The first appeals procedure, appealing an early discharge from a hospital, received a great deal of attention when Medicare's new payment system for hospitals, the prospective payment system, came into effect in 1983. Early discharges are often referred to as releasing Medicare beneficiaries from the hospital "quicker and sicker," the implication being that Medicare patients are released before they are actually ready to leave. In order to

DEPARTMENT OF HEALTH AND HUMAN SERVICES
HEALTH CARE FINANCING ADMINISTRATION

Form Approved.
OMB No. 0938-0045

REQUEST FOR RECONSIDERATION OF PART A HEALTH INSURANCE BENEFITS

INSTRUCTIONS: *Please type or print firmly.* Leave the block empty if you cannot answer it. Take or mail the WHOLE form to your Social Security office which will be glad to help you. Please read the statement on the reverse side of page 2.

1. BENEFICIARY'S NAME	2. HEALTH INSURANCE CLAIM NUMBER

3. REPRESENTATIVE'S NAME, IF APPLICABLE

(☐ RELATIVE ☐ ATTORNEY ☐ OTHER PERSON)   ☐ PROVIDER FILING

4. PLEASE ATTACH A COPY OF THE NOTICE(S) YOU RECEIVED ABOUT YOUR CLAIM TO THIS FORM.

5. THIS CLAIM IS FOR

☐ INPATIENT HOSPITAL   ☐ SKILLED NURSING FACILITY (SNF)   ☐ HEALTH MAINTENANCE ORGANIZATION (HMO)
☐ EMERGENCY HOSPITAL   ☐ HOME HEALTH AGENCY (HHA)

6. NAME AND ADDRESS OF PROVIDER (Hospital, SNF, HHA, HMO)	CITY AND STATE	PROVIDER NUMBER
7. NAME OF INTERMEDIARY	CITY AND STATE	INTERMEDIARY NUMBER

8. DATE OF ADMISSION OR START OF SERVICES	9. DATE(S) OF THE NOTICE(S) YOU RECEIVED

10. I DO NOT AGREE WITH THE DETERMINATION ON MY CLAIM. PLEASE RECONSIDER MY CLAIM BECAUSE

11. YOU MUST OBTAIN ANY EVIDENCE (For example, a letter from a doctor) YOU WISH TO SUBMIT.

☐ I HAVE ATTACHED THE FOLLOWING EVIDENCE:

☐ I WILL SEND THIS EVIDENCE WITHIN 10 DAYS:

☐ I HAVE NO ADDITIONAL EVIDENCE OR OTHER INFORMATION TO SUBMIT WITH MY CLAIM.

13. ONLY ONE SIGNATURE IS NEEDED. THIS FORM IS SIGNED BY:

☐ BENEFICIARY   ☐ REPRESENTATIVE   ☐ PROVIDER REP.

SIGN HERE ▶

14. STREET ADDRESS

12. IS THIS REQUEST FILED WITHIN 60 DAYS OF THE DATE OF YOUR NOTICE?

☐ YES   ☐ NO

IF YOU CHECKED "NO" ATTACH AN EXPLANATION OF THE REASON FOR THE DELAY TO THIS FORM.

CITY, STATE, ZIP CODE

TELEPHONE	DATE

15. If this request is signed by mark (X), TWO WITNESSES who know the person requesting reconsideration must sign in the space provided on the reverse side of this page of the form.

DO NOT FILL IN BELOW THIS LINE — FOR SOCIAL SECURITY USE — THANK YOU

16. ROUTING

☐ INTERMEDIARY

☐ HCFA, RO-MEDICARE

☐ BSS, ODR

18. SSA OR INTERMEDIARY DATE STAMP

17. ADDITIONAL INFORMATION

FORM HCFA-2649 (8-79)
DESTROY PRIOR EDITIONS

Figure 5.1   Request for Reconsideration for Part A Benefits. Form HCFA-2649.

68

REQUEST FOR HEARING
HOSPITAL INSURANCE BENEFITS PAYABLE UNDER <u>PART A</u> OF TITLE XVIII
(Amount in Controversy, $100.00 or more)
Take or mail original and all copies to your local Social Security office.

SEE
PRIVACY
ACT NOTICE
ON REVERSE
SIDE OF
FORM.

CLAIMANT	CLAIM FOR
	☐ Inpatient Hospital Services
WAGE EARNER (Leave blank if same as above)	☐ Skilled Nursing Facility Services
	☐ Home Health Agency Services
	☐ Emergency Services
HI CLAIM NUMBER	☐ Other (Identify)

NAME AND ADDRESS OF INTERMEDIARY OR PROFESSIONAL STANDARDS REVIEW ORGANIZATION	PERIOD IN QUESTION
	FROM TO
	NAME AND ADDRESS OF PROVIDER (INSTITUTION)

I disagree with the determination made on the above claim and request a hearing. My reasons for disagreement are:

Check <u>ONLY ONE</u> of the statements below:
☐ I have additional evidence to submit.
(Attach such evidence to this form or forward to the Social Security Office within 10 days.)

☐ I have <u>no</u> additional evidence to submit.

Check <u>ONLY ONE</u> of the statements below:

☐ I wish to appear in person.

☐ I do <u>not</u> wish to appear at a hearing. I request that a decision be made on the basis of the evidence in my case.

Signed by: (Either the claimant or representative should sign -- Enter addresses for both. If claimant has a representative, Form SSA-1696-U3 (Appointment of Representative) must be completed.)

SIGNATURE OR NAME OF CLAIMANT'S REPRESENTATIVE ☐ Attorney ☐ Non-Attorney	CLAIMANT'S SIGNATURE
ADDRESS	ADDRESS
CITY, STATE, AND ZIP CODE	CITY, STATE, AND ZIP CODE
AREA CODE AND TELEPHONE NUMBER	DATE:	AREA CODE AND TELEPHONE NUMBER

Claimant should not fill in below this line.

TO BE COMPLETED BY SOCIAL SECURITY ADMINISTRATION

Is this request timely filed? ☐ YES ☐ No
If "No" is checked: (1) Attach claimant's explanation for delay. (2) Attach any pertinent letter, material, or information in the Social Security Office.

Interpreter Needed _____
(Language, including sign language)

ACKNOWLEDGMENT OF REQUEST FOR HEARING
This request for hearing was filed on _____ at _____
The Administrative Law Judge will notify you of the time and place of the hearing at least 10 days in advance of the hearing.

HEARING OFFICE COPY	TO	For the Social Security Administration:
	☐ Hearing Office _____ (Location)	By _____ (Signature)
CLAIM FILE COPY	TO ☐ HCFA, Bureau of Program Operations Attn: Recon and Eval Branch Box 770, Baltimore, Md. 21203	(Title)
		(Street Address)
		(City, State, and Zip Code)
	☐ HCFA, Medicare Bureau Regional Office _____	Servicing Social Security Office Code _____

Form HA-5011-U6 (10-82)
7/81 edition may be used

ATTACH A COPY OF THE RECONSIDERATION DETERMINATION (IF AVAILABLE) TO THIS COPY

Figure 5.2   Request for a Hearing: Part A Benefits. Form HA-5011.

DEPARTMENT OF HEALTH AND HUMAN SERVICES
SOCIAL SECURITY ADMINISTRATION/OFFICE OF HEARINGS AND APPEALS

Form Approved
OMB No. 0960-0277

REQUEST FOR REVIEW OF HEARING DECISION/ORDER
(Take or mail original and all copies to your local Social Security office)

See Privacy Act
Notice on Reverse

CLAIMANT	(Check ONE) Initial Entitlement ☐ Termination or other Postentitlement Action ☐

WAGE EARNER (Leave blank if same as above)	Type Claim (Check ONE)

SOCIAL SECURITY NUMBER

Retirement or Survivors . . . . Only ☐ (RSI)
Disability, Worker or Child . . . . Only ☐ (DIWC)
Disability, Widow or Widower . . . . Only ☐ (DIWW)
Health Insurance, Part A . . . . Only ☐ (HIA)

SPOUSE'S NAME AND SOCIAL SECURITY NUMBER
(Complete ONLY in Supplemental Security Income Case)

SSI, Aged . . . . . . Only ☐ (SSIA) With Title II Claim ☐ (SSAC)
SSI, Blind . . . . . . Only ☐ (SSIB) With Title II Claim ☐ (SSBC)
SSI, Disability . . . Only ☐ (SSID) With Title II Claim ☐ (SSDC)
Other (Specify)

NAME	SSN

I disagree with the action taken on the above claim and request review of such action by the Appeals Council of the Office of Hearings and Appeals. My reasons for disagreement are:

ADDITIONAL EVIDENCE

Any additional evidence which you wish to submit must be either attached to this form or forwarded within 15 days to the Appeals Council at the address shown below. It is important that you write your Social Security number on any letter or material you send us. Where the evidence is not submitted within 15 days of this date, or within any extension of time granted by the Appeals Council, the Council will proceed to take its action based on the evidence of record.

Knowing that anyone making a false statement or representation of a material fact for use in determining the right to payment under the Social Security Act commits a crime punishable under Federal law, I certify that the above statements are true.

Signed by: (Either the claimant or representatives should sign—Enter addresses for both)

SIGNATURE OR NAME OF CLAIMANT'S REPRESENTATIVE ☐ ATTORNEY ☐ NON-ATTORNEY	CLAIMANT SIGNATURE
STREET ADDRESS	STREET ADDRESS
CITY, STATE, AND ZIP CODE	CITY, STATE, AND ZIP CODE
AREA CODE AND TELEPHONE NUMBER	DATE	AREA CODE AND TELEPHONE NUMBER

Claimant should not fill in below this line

TO BE COMPLETED BY SOCIAL SECURITY ADMINISTRATION

Is this request filed timely? ☐ Yes ☐ No

If "NO" is checked: (1) attach claimant's explanation for delay;
(2) attach any pertinent letter, material or information in Social Security Office.

ACKNOWLEDGEMENT OF RECEIPT OF REQUEST FOR REVIEW OF HEARING DECISION/ORDER

This request for Review of Hearing Decision/Order was filed on _____ at _____
The APPEALS COUNCIL will notify you of its action on your request.

For the Social Security Administration.

APPEALS COUNCIL
OFFICE OF HEARINGS AND APPEALS, SSA
P.O. BOX 3200
ARLINGTON, VA 22203

SIGNATURE BY:

TITLE

STREET ADDRESS

CITY

STATE	ZIP CODE

SERVICING SOCIAL SECURITY OFFICE CODE

Form HA-520-U5 (6/88)
Destroy old stock

Figure 5.3   Request for Social Security Appeals Council Review. Form HA-520.

understand the right to appeal an early discharge it is first necessary to explain DRGs and the prospective payment system.

One of the most frequently asked questions about Medicare is, "What are DRGs?" DRG stands for Diagnostic Related Group. According to the patient's diagnosis, he or she is assigned one of 477 DRG codes when entering the hospital. The hospital is reimbursed for the patient's care based upon the predetermined amount for that code. Tables 5.1 and 5.2 show the major diagnostic categories DRGs fall under and the top ten DRGs in 1987.

The DRG method of reimbursement is called the prospective payment system (PPS). The system has the effect of a cap or limit on the amount of money that hospitals receive from Medicare. If the hospital's actual costs fall under the cap, it gets to keep 50

Table 5.1   Major Diagnostic Categories Used in Medicare's Payment System

(Medicare's 477 DRGs Fall within These 23 Categories)

1. Nervous System Diseases and Disorders
2. Eye Diseases and Disorders
3. Ear, Nose, and Throat Diseases and Disorders
4. Respiratory System Diseases and Disorders
5. Circulatory System Diseases and Disorders
6. Digestive System Diseases and Disorders
7. Hepatobiliary System and Pancreas Diseases and Disorders
8. Musculoskeletal System and Corrective Tissue Diseases
9. Skin, Subcutaneous Tissue, and Breast Diseases
10. Endocrine, Nutritional, and Metabolic Diseases
11. Kidney and Urinary Tract Diseases and Disorders
12. Male Reproductive System Diseases and Disorders
13. Female Reproductive System Diseases and Disorders
14. Pregnancy, Childbirth, and the Puerperium
15. Normal Newborns and Conditions in Perinatal Period
16. Blood, Blood-Forming Organs, and Immunity Diseases and Disorders
17. Myeloproliterative Disorders and Poorly Differentiated Malignancy, Other Neoplasms
18. Infectious and Parasitic Diseases
19. Mental Disorders
20. Substance Use and Substance-Induced Organic Disorders
21. Injury, Poisoning, and Toxic Effect of Drugs
22. Burns
23. Selected Factors Influencing Health Status

Source: U.S. House of Representatives, Background Material and Data on Programs within the Jurisdiction of the Committee on Ways and Means, Washington, DC, 1989.

percent of the difference up to a maximum of 5 percent of the cap. If the hospital's costs are greater, it loses money. Adjusted payments are made to hospitals serving a disproportionately large number of low-income and severely ill Medicare patients and for patients with extraordinarily long stays in a hospital (the latter are called outliers). At this writing the DRG system does not apply to psychiatric, rehabilitative, pediatric, and long-term-care hospitals or units of hospitals.

The reason DRGs are important is that Congress adopted the DRG system to encourage hospitals to provide quality care *in the least amount of time.* Under the prospective payment system hospitals have a financial incentive to release individuals as soon as possible to reduce health-care costs. However, hospitals also cannot discharge patients before they are "ready." Medicare statutes require *all* hospitals to give each Medicare beneficiary a written statement concerning his or her rights to care, the right to appeal denials of benefits, and potential liability for care at or about the time of hospital admission. (See page 64.)

When Medicare patients are hospitalized they have the following rights:

The right to receive all the hospital care that is necessary for the proper diagnosis and treatment of the illness and

Table 5.2   Top Ten Diagnostic Related Groups (DRGs) with the Most Discharges

1. Heart Failure and Shock (DRG number 127)
2. Angina Pectoris (DRG number 140)
3. Specific Cerebrovascular Disorders except Transient Ischemic Attacks (DRG number 014)
4. Simple Pneumonia and Pleurisy (DRG number 089)
5. Esophagitis, Gastroentiritis, and Miscellaneous Digestive Disorders (DRG number 182)
6. Bronchitis and Asthma (DRG number 096)
7. Major Joint Procedures (DRG number 209)
8. Nutritional and Miscellaneous Metabolic Disorders (DRG number 296)
9. Cardiac Arrythmia and Conduction Disorders (DRG number 138)
10. Transient Ischemic Attacks (DRG number 015)

Source: U.S. House of Representatives, Background Material and Data on Programs within the Jurisdiction of the Committee on Ways and Means, Washington, DC, 1989. Data are for 1987.

injury. *According to federal law, the discharge date must be determined solely by medical need, not by DRGs or Medicare payments.*

The right to be fully informed about decisions affecting the patient's Medicare coverage, payment for the hospital stay, and any post-hospital services.

The right to request a review by a Peer Review Organization of any written Notice of Noncoverage received from the hospital stating that Medicare will no longer pay for the hospital care.

Appealing an Early Discharge from the Hospital

Taking these rights into account, sometimes a hospital's Utilization Review Committee (URC), which is responsible for reviewing a hospital's cases, may decide to discharge a patient before he or she is ready to leave. When this happens the Medicare patient has the right to appeal the decision with the local Peer Review Organization (PRO). The PRO monitors the prospective payment system. Formerly referred to as PSROs, PROs are organizations in each state selected and paid by the federal government to review hospital treatment of Medicare patients. They are also the bodies that oversee the Medicare appeals process for hospitals.

There are two situations involving an early discharge that a beneficiary may want to appeal. They occur when the physician and hospital agree and when the physician and hospital do not agree on the decision to discharge.

When the Physician and Hospital Agree

Usually when a patient is discharged from a hospital the physician and hospital are in agreement with the decision. The following appeals process applies in this situation:

The patient receives a "Notice of Noncoverage" including instructions on how to appeal. He or she is liable for all hospital costs after 48 hours.

The patient has until noon of the first working day after receiving the notice to request an immediate review of the case. Acting quickly and requesting an immediate review is the only way to delay having to leave the hospital and to get a quick response back from the PRO. Otherwise the PRO has 30 days to respond, and the beneficiary will have to leave the hospital before a decision has been made on the appeal.

The PRO then must notify the patient of its review decision no later than one full working day after receiving the review request and records.

If the PRO agrees with the original decision, the patient becomes liable for costs beginning at noon of the day after the PRO's decision. The beneficiary should make sure that the hospital submits the bill to Medicare so he or she can continue an appeal.

When the Hospital and PRO Agree but the Physician Doesn't

In some cases the hospital and the PRO will agree that a notice of noncoverage is appropriate, but the physician does not agree and this is stated on the notice. In this case all of the rules above apply except that the PRO can take up to three days to complete its review. The patient is liable for costs beginning with the third calendar day after receiving the original notice of noncoverage, even if the PRO has not completed its decision.

In both cases, when the physician is or is not in agreement with the hospital, if the beneficiary does not request a review immediately upon receiving a notice of noncoverage the patient still has up to 60 days to ask for reconsideration, and the PRO then has 30 days to reconsider.

The following sections describe the nine other major areas of Medicare appeals.

Preadmission Notice of Noncoverage by a Hospital

Sometimes Medicare beneficiaries are refused admission to a hospital because the hospital's Utilization Review Committee has decided that it is not necessary for the beneficiary to receive hospital care. The patient is then liable for all costs, if he or she insists on being admitted. The following rules apply in this situation:

The beneficiary must be notified in writing of the reasons for the preadmission denial.

The patient has three days to request, in writing, an expedited reconsideration from the PRO. The doctor's support will help considerably in this case. The PRO has three days to respond. If the beneficiary does not submit the request in three days, the PRO has 30 days to respond. (The patient has a maximum of 60 days to make the request.)

Hospital Notice of Noncoverage for Admission That Was Not Medically Necessary

Some beneficiaries may be admitted to the hospital and then receive notice that the admission was not necessary. If the hospital's Utilization Review Committee determines that admission was not medically necessary, it can issue a notice of noncoverage. The steps to follow in this situation are the same as those for early discharges from hospitals.

Notice of Noncoverage as Part of an "Automatic" Retrospective Review by the PRO

Even after a patient has been discharged from the hospital, he or she can receive a notice from Medicare that the stay is not covered. This situation occurs when the PRO conducts an automatic review of hospital stays, which is part of its responsibilities, and, in the review, decides that a particular stay was not appropriate. Usually the beneficiary is not responsible for any charges, as there was no way of knowing that the stay would not be covered. This is called a "waiver of liability." However, in some cases the beneficiary is liable. A common example is when a beneficiary has received a Notice of Noncoverage from another hospital for the same reasons that he or she was admitted for the hospital stay under question. Either the hospital or the Medicare beneficiary can appeal a retrospective review by the PRO. However, only a beneficiary, not a hospital, can continue the appeal beyond the PRO's reconsideration.

Denial of Skilled-Nursing-Facility Services, Home Health Services, and Hospice Care

In most cases, appealing one of these procedures is well worth the trouble, particularly if a beneficiary has been denied skilled-nursing-facility services or home health care. Unfortunately, it is often the case that the beneficiary who is in need of and denied either service is also too sick to appeal a denial. In this case it might be appropriate for an advocate for the beneficiary to step in and appeal in his or her behalf, particularly if the patient's physician agrees that the care is needed.

Often skilled-nursing facilities and home health agencies do not submit claims if they anticipate that Medicare will not pay. However, as mentioned previously, the beneficiary has the right to request that the facility or agency submit a "no-payment billing." Under a recent federal court decision, *Sarassat v. Bowen*, all skilled-nursing facilities must give patients written notice whenever they determine that the beneficiary's medical condition doesn't meet Medicare's guidelines. The notice must inform the beneficiary of the right to have a claim submitted and to appeal an unfavorable decision.

Reconsideration for skilled-nursing facilities, home health care, and hospice services are submitted to the fiscal intermediary or local Social Security office.

Part B Appeals

Denial of a Usually Covered Doctor's Visit or Other Service

Medicare Part B carriers notify beneficiaries of their determination on claims in written notices called Explanation of Medicare Benefits (EOMBs). (See Figure 4.6.) Sometimes an EOMB states that a service is not covered. If the beneficiary does not agree with this decision he or she can file a Part B appeal. Here are some of the reasons Part B claims are denied:

The service was not considered reasonable and necessary

Too many visits were made to a provider such as a physician for a service

Ambulance service was not necessary

Durable medical equipment is not considered necessary

Duplication of services

Physical therapy that is no longer needed for recovery from an acute condition but is considered maintenance

A billing error

The carrier considers the service as one excluded from Medicare, such as eyeglasses or dental care

There are often good reasons to file Part B appeals. The following rules apply:

After receipt of the EOMB stating that a service has not been covered, the beneficiary should request the Medicare carrier to review its decision. The request may be made in the form of a letter or by using Form HCFA-1964. (See Figure 5.4.) The EOMB must be attached, and the request must be filed within six months of the date of receipt of the EOMB. To strengthen the appeal, the following should be included:

Letters from physicians stating why the service was needed

Medical records

Orders and prescriptions

Medicare records (federal law permits access to Part B carriers' records)

A review generally takes 45 days but can take longer. If the carrier has determined that partial payment of the claim is being allowed, the beneficiary will receive a letter describing the action. If the claim is being paid in full, the beneficiary will receive an EOMB.

If the patient is not satisfied with the decision and the amount in question is over $100, the next step is to request a Medicare-carrier hearing, which will be conducted by a hearing officer who is employed by the carrier. (When the case involves less than

DEPARTMENT OF HEALTH AND HUMAN SERVICES
HEALTH CARE FINANCING ADMINISTRATION

Form Approved
OMB No. 0938-0033

REQUEST FOR REVIEW OF PART B MEDICARE CLAIM
Medical Insurance Benefits - Social Security Act

NOTICE—Anyone who misrepresents or falsifies essential information requested by this form may upon conviction be subject to fine and imprisonment under Federal Law.

1 Carrier's Name and Address

2 Name of Patient

3 Health Insurance Claim Number

4 I do not agree with the determination you made on my claim as described on my Explanation of Medicare

Benefits dated:

5 MY REASONS ARE: (Attach a copy of the Explanation of Medicare Benefits, or describe the service, date of service, and physician's name—NOTE.—If the date on the Notice of Benefits mentioned in item 3 is more than six months ago, include your reason for not making this request earlier.)

6 Describe Illness or Injury:

7 ☐ I have additional evidence to submit. (Attach such evidence to this form.)

☐ I do not have additional evidence.

COMPLETE ALL OF THE INFORMATION REQUESTED. SIGN AND RETURN THE FIRST COPY AND ANY ATTACHMENTS TO THE CARRIER NAMED ABOVE. IF YOU NEED HELP, TAKE THIS AND YOUR NOTICE FROM THE CARRIER TO A SOCIAL SECURITY OFFICE, OR TO THE CARRIER. KEEP THE DUPLICATE COPY OF THIS FORM FOR YOUR RECORDS.

8 SIGNATURE OF **EITHER** THE CLAIMENT **OR** HIS REPRESENTATIVE

Representative	Claimant
Address	Address
City, State, and ZIP Code	City, State, and ZIP Code
Telephone Number Date	Telephone Number Date

Form HCFA-1964 (8-85)

(over)

Figure 5.4   Request for Review of Part B Medicare Claim. Form HCFA-1964.

$100 there is no further recourse at this point. However, claims may be combined to reach the $100 amount.) The request may be made by writing a letter to the person who signed the review or to Medicare Communications or by filling out Form HCFA-1965. (See Figure 5.5.)

At least 14 days before the hearing is to take place, the beneficiary is notified of the date, time, and place of the hearing. The hearing may be by phone. Someone else may represent the beneficiary, in which case the beneficiary must sign a statement agreeing to the representation or fill out Form SSA-1696. (See Figure 5.6.)

The next three steps are essentially the same as steps 2, 3, and 4 of Part A appeals. If at least $500 is in controversy, the beneficiary may request a hearing from an administrative law judge employed by the Social Security Administration. Then he or she may request a review by the Social Security Appeals Council and then by the Federal District Court. These steps are described in the preceding section on Medicare Part A appeals.

New Information Becomes Available

A case may be reopened up to 12 months after the final appeals process when new information such as a processing error may shed new light on the appeal. Extensions may be made under special circumstances. In cases of fraud there is a four-year limit.

Getting a Lower Medicare Payment than Expected for a Physician's Service or Other Part B Claim

If the approved charge on the EOMB is more than 30 percent below the doctor's actual charge, the beneficiary should request a review. To file an appeal, the procedures described above should be used.

Part A and Part B Appeals

Denial of Eligibility for Medicare

An applicant who is denied eligibility for Medicare has the right to know why. To appeal a denial of Medicare eligibility, the applicant must submit a written appeal along with any documents

DEPARTMENT OF HEALTH AND HUMAN SERVICES
HEALTH CARE FINANCING ADMINISTRATION

Form Approved
OMB No. 66-R0044

REQUEST FOR HEARING - PART B MEDICARE CLAIM
Medical Insurance Benefits - Social Security Act

NOTICE—Anyone who misrepresents or falsifies essential information requested by this form may upon conviction be subject to fine and imprisonment under Federal Law.

Carrier's Name and Address	**1** Name of Patient
	2 Health Insurance Claim Number

3 I disagree with the review determination on my claim, and request a hearing before a hearing officer of the insurance carrier named above.

MY REASONS ARE: *(Attach a copy of the Review Notice. NOTE.—If the review decision was made more than 6 months ago include your reason for not making this request earlier)*

4 Check one of the Following:

☐ I have additional evidence to submit.
(Attach such evidence to this form or forward it to the carrier within 10 days.)

☐ I do not have additional evidence.

Check <u>Only One</u> of the Statements Below:

☐ I wish to appear in person before the Hearing Officer.

☐ I do not wish to appear and hereby request a decision on the evidence before the Hearing Officer.

5 EITHER THE CLAIMANT OR REPRESENTATIVE SHOULD SIGN IN THE APPROPRIATE SPACE BELOW:

Signature or Name of Claimant's Representative ➡	Claimant's Signature ➡
Address	Address
City, State, and ZIP Code	City, State, and ZIP Code
Telephone Number / Date	Telephone Number / Date

(Claimant should not write below this line)

ACKNOWLEDGMENT OF REQUEST FOR HEARING

Your request for a hearing was received on _____. You will be notified of the time and place of the hearing at least 10 days before the date of the hearing.

Signed	Date

Form **HCFA-1965** (8-79) (Formerly SSA-1965)

Figure 5.5   Request for Medicare-Carrier Hearing. Form HCFA-1965.

DEPARTMENT OF
HEALTH AND HUMAN SERVICES
SOCIAL SECURITY ADMINISTRATION

| NAME (Claimant) (Print or Type) | SOCIAL SECURITY NUMBER |
| WAGE EARNER (if different) | SOCIAL SECURITY NUMBER |

Section I APPOINTMENT OF REPRESENTATIVE

I appoint this individual _____
(Name and Address)

to act as my representative in connection with my claim or asserted right under:

☐ Title II (RSDI) ☐ Title XVI (SSI) ☐ Title IV FMSHA (Black Lung) ☐ Title XVIII (Medicare Coverage)

I authorize this individual to make or give any request or notice; to present or elicit evidence; to obtain information; and to receive any notice in connection with my pending claim or asserted right wholly in my stead.

SIGNATURE (Claimant)	ADDRESS
TELEPHONE NUMBER	DATE
(Area Code)	

Section II ACCEPTANCE OF APPOINTMENT

I, _____ , hereby accept the above appointment. I certify that I have not been suspended or prohibited from practice before the Social Security Administration; that I am not, as a current or former officer or employee of the United States, disqualified from acting as the claimant's representative; and that I will not charge or receive any fee for the representation unless it has been authorized in accordance with the laws and regulations referred to on the reverse side hereof. In the event that I decide not to charge or collect a fee for the representation, I will notify the Social Security Administration. (Completion of Section III satisfies this requirement.)

I am a / an _____
(Attorney, union representative, relative, law student, etc.)

SIGNATURE (Representative)	ADDRESS
TELEPHONE NUMBER	DATE
(Area code)	

Section III (Optional) WAIVER OF FEE

I waive my right to charge and collect a fee under Section 206 of the Social Security Act, and I release my client (the claimant) from any obligations, contractual or otherwise, which may be owed to me for services I have performed in connection with my client's claim or asserted right.

| SIGNATURE (Representative) | DATE |

WAIVER OF DIRECT PAYMENT

I ONLY waive my right to direct certification of a fee from the withheld past-due benefits of my client (the claimant). I do NOT, however, waive my right to petition for and be authorized to charge and collect a fee directly from my client.

| SIGNATURE (Representative) | DATE |

Form SSA-1696-U4 (3-88)   *(See Important Information on Reverse)*
Detroy prior editions

Figure 5.6   Agreement To Have Representation at Hearing. Form SSA-1696.

Figure 5.6   (continued)

HOW TO COMPLETE THIS FORM

Print or type your full name and your Social Security number.

Section I — APPOINTMENT OF REPRESENTATIVE

You may appoint as your representative an attorney or any other qualified individual. You may appoint more than one person, but see "The Fee You Owe The Representative(s)." You may NOT appoint as your representative an organization, the law firm, a group, etc. Example, you go to a law firm or legal aid group for help with your claim, you may appoint any attorney or other qualified individual from that firm or group, but NOT the firm or group itself.

Check the block(s) for the program in which you have a claim. Title II, check if your claim concerns disability or retirement benefits, etc. Title XVI, check if the claim concerns Supplemental Security Income (SSI) payments. Title IV FMSHA (Federal Mine Safety and Health Act), check if the claim is for black lung benefits. Title XVIII, check only in connection with a proceeding before the Social Security Administration involving entitlement to medicare coverage or enrollment in the supplementary medical insurance plan (SMIP). More than one block may be checked.

Section II — ACCEPTANCE OF APPOINTMENT

The individual whom you appoint in Section I above, completes this part. Completion of this section is desirable in all cases, but it is mandatory only if the appointed individual is not an attorney.

Section III (Optional) — WAIVER OF FEE

This section may be completed by your representative if he/she will not charge any fee for services performed in this claim. If you had appointed a co-counsel (second representative) in Section I and he/she will also not charge you a fee, then the co-counsel should also sign this section or give a separate waiver statement.

GENERAL INFORMATION

1. When you have a representative:

   We will deal directly with your representative on all matters that affect your claim. Occasionally, with the permission of your representative, we may deal directly with you on specific issues. We will rely on your representative to keep you informed on the status of your claim, but you may contact us directly for any information about your claim.

2. The authority of your representative:

   Your representative has the authority to act totally on your behalf. This means he/she can (1) obtain information about your claim the same as you; (2) submit evidence; (3) make statements about facts and provisions of the law; and (4) make any request (including a fee request). It is important, therefore, that you are represented by a qualified individual.

3. When will the representation stop:

   We will stop recognizing or dealing with your representative when (1) you tell us that he/she is no longer your representative; (2) your representative does any one of the following: (a) submits a fee petition, or (b) tells us that he/she is withdrawing from the claim, or (c) he/she violates any on our rules and regulations, and a hearing is held before an administrative law judge (designated as hearing officer) who orders your representative disqualified or suspended as a representative of any Social Security claimant.

4. The fee you owe the representative(s):

   Every representative you appoint has a right to petition for a fee. To charge you a fee, a representative must first file a fee petition with us. Irrespective of your fee agreement, you never owe more than the fee we have authorized in a written notice to you and your representative(s). (Out-of-pocket expenses are not included). If your claim went to court, you may owe an additional fee for your representative's services before the court.

5. How we determine the fee:

   We use the criteria on the back of the fee petition (Form SSA 1560-U4), a copy of which your representative must send you.

6. Review of the fee authorization:

   If you or your representative disagrees with the fee authorization, either of you may request a review. Instructions for filing this review are on the fee authorization notice.

7. Payment of fees:

   If past-due benefits are payable in your claim, we generally withhold 25 percent of the past-due benefits toward possible attorney fees. If no past-due benefits are payable or this is an SSI claim, then payment of the fee we have authorized is your responsibility.

8. Penalty for charging an unauthorized fee:

   If your representative wants to charge and collect from you a fee that is greater than what we had authorized, then he/she is in violation of the law and regulations. Promptly report this to your nearest Social Security office.

supporting the case. This must be done within 60 days after the written notice of denial. The case will be reviewed by SSA staff, who in turn will inform the beneficiary of the decision on the appeal and any further appeals rights.

Denial of "Waiver of Beneficiary Liability" in Noncoverage Situations

As discussed earlier, there are times when a beneficiary does not know, and could not be expected to know, that certain services do not meet Medicare's guidelines. A "waiver of liability" refers to releasing the beneficiary from the responsibility to pay for services under these circumstances. Part B waivers apply when the following were not known, or could not be expected to be known, by the beneficiary:

When the service that was performed was not "reasonable and necessary"

When the service was "custodial" in nature

When a service was not being provided under strict Medicare definition

As a general rule, when a patient receives a notice that Medicare is not covering certain Part A charges, he or she usually does not have to pay anything. For Part B claims, Medicare first notifies the physician that coverage is denied. At this point physicians who did not accept assignment on the claim must refund the patient's payment. Here are the basic rules that apply to waiver-of-liability appeals:

Most waiver-of-liability appeals are begun by providers, but a patient can request a review. A hospital's appeal is limited to a decision from the PRO. Only a beneficiary can continue a Part A appeal.

If the patient is requesting the review, it is most important to submit convincing evidence that he or she could not have known that Medicare would not cover the services in question.

Part A appeals should first be made to the PRO or fiscal intermediary. Part B appeals should be made to the Medicare carrier.

Chapter 6

Supplementing Medicare

FACTS ON SUPPLEMENTAL INSURANCE

- Eighty-two percent of older health consumers have chosen a medigap insurance policy to supplement their Medicare coverage.

- In 1989 premiums for medigap policies ranged from $192 to $1,320 per policyholder. The most popular policies cost from $420 to $600 a year.

- Most policies that are called Medicare supplements *cover services only after Medicare pays first*. As a general rule if Medicare does not pay, neither will the Medicare supplement.

- The Health Insurance Association of America estimates that 15 percent of all supplemental-policy customers have more than one policy.

- Health maintenance organizations (HMOs), which generally provide care at less expense to the consumer than traditional fee-for-service care, are a relatively new option for Medicare beneficiaries.

- There are now more than 150 Medicare health maintenance organizations providing services to 1.1 million Medicare beneficiaries.

- Medicaid is a public-assistance program that pays for medical care for low-income persons. Ten percent of Medicare beneficiaries are also covered by Medicaid. Persons with Medicaid do not need supplemental insurance.

- Older persons with low incomes may qualify for a "Medicaid buy in," in which Medicaid will pay for Medicare's premium and at least some of the deductibles and copayments.

Introduction

Chapter 1 pointed out that Medicare is a double-edged sword: while it provides access to health care for 97 percent of older adults, it covers only about 40 percent of their total health costs. Because of Medicare's limitations it is necessary for beneficiaries to supplement the program. This chapter covers 11 options for filling in Medicare's gaps. Some of these options, such as purchasing medigap policies and joining health maintenance organizations (HMOs), make great sense for Medicare beneficiaries. Others, such as covering costs out of pocket or purchasing indemnity insurance, are bad choices but are mentioned here as warnings.

Several of the supplemental options are relatively new to older adults. For example, until recently HMOs had difficulty getting reimbursed for services to Medicare recipients, and they were not a viable alternative for seniors. And although the Medicare Catastrophic Coverage Act of 1988 was repealed, an important provision of the law remained called the "Medicaid buy in," which helps pay some of the expenses of low-income Medicare recipients. However, as of this writing the benefit is so new that many states have not yet started their "buy in" programs.

Here are the 11 major options for supplementing Medicare:

1. Covering out-of-pocket health-care costs

2. Continuing group health insurance

3. Receiving coverage from an employer

4. Purchasing supplemental health insurance

5. Joining a health maintenance organization

6. Joining a Preferred Provider Organization

7. Becoming eligible for Medicaid

8. Taking advantage of the government's new low-income Medicaid "buy in"

9. Taking advantage of Department of Veterans Affairs (VA) benefits

10. Purchasing catastrophic or major medical insurance

11. Purchasing indemnity and other policies

Covering Out-of-Pocket Health-Care Costs

Some people may feel that they are able to cover all their health-care expenses out of their own pockets after age 65. However, it is important to keep in mind that the cost of medical care has increased almost twice as fast as the costs of other goods and services in the past decade. Thus, personal resources that are adequate today may not be so a couple of years from now.

Continuing Group Health Insurance

When possible, the best way to supplement Medicare is to continue group-health-insurance coverage from work or a professional or fraternal organization. The ability to continue health-insurance coverage is a common provision among the majority of employer plans. Of those older Americans with supplemental insurance, about 36 percent receive it as a retirement benefit. And in 1985, 72 percent of workers who participated in employer plans continued coverage after early retirement, while 66 percent had coverage continued after retirement at age 65.

Thanks to a 1985 law, many Americans who would have lost their group health insurance because of unemployment, divorce, or the death or retirement of a spouse are now able to keep their coverage. Individuals have to pay both the employer and employee portions of the premium, however, plus a 2 percent administrative fee. The following are eligible to continue their current group health insurance for at least 36 months:

The widow or widower or divorced spouse of a worker

The Medicare-ineligible spouse of a retiring worker

In addition, workers and their spouses who have been laid off or terminated (except for gross misconduct) or are working reduced hours (the new law does not apply to workers employed by a company with fewer than 20 workers) may continue coverage for 18 months.

Coverage for Age 65-plus Workers

There are a number of advantages to working past age 65, one of which is the availability of group health insurance. Employers with 20 or more employees are required by law to offer the same health benefits to workers and spouses 65 or older that they offer to younger workers. The worker who is 65 or older has the option of accepting or rejecting the health plan. Companies are not allowed to offer Medicare supplemental coverage to older workers who reject the employer's general health plan.

Purchasing Supplemental Health Insurance

According to the Health Insurance Association of America, 78 percent of older health consumers have chosen a medigap insurance policy to supplement their Medicare coverage. The purpose of Medicare supplemental policies is to fill in the gaps that Medicare does not cover. Policies that are called Medicare supplements generally *cover services only after Medicare pays first*. If Medicare denies payment for services, the Medicare supplement also will not pay for those services.

Private insurance for health-care costs is not a new idea but has been prominent since World War II. However, until passage of Medicare in 1965 coverage for older adults was not workable for insurance companies because of the high rates of illness for this age group. After passage of Medicare, though, the risks for private insurance companies were greatly reduced, because they could issue policies that simply picked up some of the costs that Medicare did not cover.

In general, companies offering supplemental-health-insurance policies to seniors do not offer plans that do more than build upon what Medicare covers. Most plans cover copayments and deductibles. Some limited policies add extra benefits, but they also cost more. In brief, it is very difficult to find and afford a policy that covers long-term care, prescription drugs, and physician costs that are more than Medicare's approved rate.

Regulations governing Medicare supplements vary a great deal by state. For example, in Massachusetts older residents have three basic policies to choose from, while older Coloradans have more than 90. Eligibility requirements also vary a great deal.

Premiums for supplemental coverage reflect the comprehensiveness of the package, as well as administrative and marketing costs that are from 15 to 35 percent of the premium. In 1989 premiums ranged from $192 to $1,320 per policyholder. The most popular policies cost from $420 to $600 a year. Early in 1990 the Blue Cross/Blue Shield Association estimated that premiums would increase from 20 to 76 percent as a result of inflation and repeal of the Medicare Catastrophic Coverage Act.

Minimum Standards for Insurance Policies

There are minimum standards that policies must meet to be labeled Medicare supplements. They apply only to policies issued after 1980 and they do *not* apply to other policies such as long-term-care insurance or hospital indemnity coverage. These standards are often referred to by the amendment to the Social Security law that set the standards, the Baucus Amendment (named for a senator from Montana, Democrat Max Baucus). No policy may be sold as a Medicare supplement unless it meets these standards. Forty-six states meet or exceed the minimum requirements—the other four states are subject to federal certification of policies. In addition, in 1990 the National Association of Insurance Commissioners adopted a standard that all *new* policies must provide a $75 deductible on Part B rather than the previously allowed deductible of up to $200. Older consumers should consult their insurance commissions (see page 173) to learn what standards apply in their states. Unfortunately, as a recent article in *Consumer Reports* magazine points out, the Baucus Amendment generally is not enforced by the states.

The following are the standards set forth by the 1980 Baucus Amendment:

1. Policies must supplement both Medicare Part A and Part B. For Part A, policies must cover the hospital copayment for days 61–90 and for all lifetime reserve

days, as well as cover 90 percent of hospital expenses for 365 days after all Medicare benefits are exhausted. For Part B, the Baucus Amendment requires a Medicare supplemental policy to cover the 20 percent of the Medicare-approved charges for which the senior is responsible.

2. No preexisting condition may be excluded for more than six months.

3. The policyholder must be allowed a ten-day "free look" with cancellation rights for a policy purchased from an agent or 30 days for a policy purchased through the mail.

4. Supplemental policies are required to have minimum loss ratios of 60 percent on individual policies and 75 percent on group coverage.

5. Misleading sales practices are prohibited. Penalties will be handed down to companies or agents that fraudulently misrepresent themselves as agents of the federal government in order to sell Medicare supplements, or knowingly sell duplicate coverage that does not pay in addition to existing benefits. Conviction for these offenses could result in fines of up to $25,000, or up to five years' imprisonment, or both.

6. When replacement of one policy with another occurs, the agent must give the consumer a "Notice to Applicant Regarding Replacement Insurance" to sign. The agent is required to give one copy to the consumer and to send another to the home office.

7. The agent must give the consumer an Outline of Coverage and a Buyer's Guide as a disclosure of policy benefits.

In addition, the National Association of Insurance Commissioners (NAIC) adopted the following Consumer Protection Amendments on December 7, 1989. It is expected that most states will have adopted these standards by the end of 1990.

1. All policies must be guaranteed renewable.

2. Specific limitations will be imposed on agent commissions to eliminate "churning," the inappropriate replacing of an existing policy with a new one.

3. Agents must give the "Notice to Applicant Regarding Replacement Insurance" mentioned above. In addition, agents and companies must ask certain questions about Medicare and the applicant's current coverage in order to garner information about whether the sale of a Medicare supplement policy is appropriate.

4. Companies must establish standards for marketing and procedures for verifying compliance. In addition, high pressure and other deceptive sales practices are prohibited.

5. The sale of more than one Medicare supplemental policy is prohibited except under very limited circumstances when the additional policy insures no more than 100 percent of the individual's actual medical expenses under the combined policies.

6. Agents must report to the State Insurance Department those individuals who have in force more than one policy.

7. Preexisting condition clauses must *not* be included in any replacement policy. Waiting periods, elimination periods, and probationary periods are also prohibited.

Regulation of Supplemental Health Insurance

The sale of supplemental health insurance is regulated by state insurance commissions. When state guidelines are not as stringent as those set out above, the federal Department of Health and Human Services determines whether policies sold in those states meet federal guidelines.

A recent study by the General Accounting Office (GAO) found that most large commercial carriers with premiums of $50 million or more met the loss-ratio requirements of the law (see above). This is important, because these are the carriers from which consumers are most likely to purchase insurance. For example, the loss ratios of Blue Cross/Blue Shield and Prudential Life Insurance were 81.1 and 77.9, respectively, in 1984. However, GAO reported one alarming finding: of the 142 policies studied, *most* were below the Baucus Amendment's cost-ratio targets.

Types of Medicare Supplemental Policies

There are three basic types of Medicare supplemental policies.

Thrifty Models provide minimal coverage required by law.

Standard Models provide minimal coverage plus coverage of the Part A deductible. They also might offer extras such as private-duty nursing, foreign travel, and extra skilled-nursing-facility days. They might also cover 30 to 50 percent of the non-Medicare-covered Part B charges. Such a policy might read, "pays 120 percent of each Medicare approved charge."

Deluxe Models are expensive and generally require potential policyholders to fill out a health questionnaire. These policies will cover Part B expenses above Medicare's approved charges. Some of these policies also cover a portion of prescription drugs.

Common Health Insurance Practices

Health-insurance policies are legal contracts that employ precise legal language and can be confusing. Here are some important supplemental-policy features that older health consumers should check when shopping for Medicare supplemental insurance. There are many checklists available for comparing these features. Often state insurance commissions or offices on aging make them available to seniors. In addition, several books on the market offer excellent checklists. (See Part Two.)

The *deductible* is an initial amount of health expenses that the individual must pay before any expenses are reimbursed by the plan (such as Medicare Part B's $75 deductible). The deductible must be satisfied generally every calendar year, although many plans have three-month carryover provisions in which the last three months of the previous year can be applied toward satisfaction of the following year's deductible.

The *coinsurance* amount *(copayment)* is based on the idea that the individual and the insurance company share the cost of a medical expense. The plan participant pays a portion of the recognized medical expenses, and the plan pays the remaining portion. *Medicare supplemental policies are required to pay the 20 percent coinsurance amount that Medicare does not pay. They are not required to pay the excess amount.*

Because meeting the coinsurance and deductible amounts can pose a hardship, most plans contain a *limit on out-of-pocket expenditures.* Once an individual has reached the maximum, say $5,000, covered expenses are reimbursed in full for the remainder of the year. The limit is usually renewed at the start of the calendar year for each individual participant.

Preexisting condition clauses restrict payment for health problems an individual had prior to becoming insured.

Exclusions will not pay benefits for an illness arising from that condition.

Waiting periods will not pay for a preexisting condition until after the policyholder has had the policy for a specified period of time. The 1989 NAIC amendments prohibit waiting periods in Medicare supplemental policies.

Benefit maximums limit the amount a policy will pay for a given benefit. A benefit can be a length of time or a dollar amount.

Lifetime maximums are upper limits on the total benefits a policy will ever pay. The lifetime maximum is commonly quite high— $250,000 or $1 million, for example.

Conditions of renewability are one of the most important policy features. According to NAIC's 1989 standards, all Medicare supplemental policies must be guaranteed renewable. The company agrees to continue insuring the individual up to a certain age as long as he or she pays the premium. Companies cannot raise premiums unless they are raised for an entire class of policyholders, such as everyone in a geographical area with the same kind of policy. Some plans are guaranteed renewable for life.

The *A.M. Best rating* analyzes the financial stability of insurance companies. An A+ is the highest rating a company can attain.

Shopping Tips for Supplemental Health Insurance

Here are important guidelines that older health consumers should follow when shopping for supplemental health insurance. Some guidelines have been adapted from recommendations made by the Health Care Financing Administration, which runs the Medicare program.

- Review Medicare's gaps to determine what is important in a Medicare supplement. Give special consideration to the amount that a policy will pay above 20 percent of Medicare's approved charge. Also consider the policy features listed above, such as premiums and maximum benefit clauses.

- Work with agents and companies that have good reputations in the community.

- Talk with friends who have good claims experience. As a general rule, one comprehensive policy is all that is needed. The Health Insurance Association of America estimates that 15 percent of all supplemental policyholders currently have more than one policy.

- Beware of replacing existing coverage. Be suspicious of a suggestion to give up a policy and buy a replacement.

- Watch out for charlatans. Policies to supplement Medicare are neither sold nor serviced by state or federal governments. Anyone pretending to be from Medicare or any other government agency is subject to penalties. Anyone suggesting that they are selling insurance through a government-sponsored program should be reported to a state division of insurance.

- Don't pay cash for insurance. Write a check or money order payable to the company, not the agent.

- Keep the agent's and/or company's names, addresses, and telephone numbers.

- Any agent knowingly trying to sell policies that duplicate Medicare coverage or other private insurance (unless it pays duplicate benefits) is subject to criminal penalties.

- Group insurance sold by associations is only sometimes a good buy. In addition, beware of companies that pretend to be well-known seniors' organizations. For example, the California Insurance Department has ordered the National Association of Retired Persons (NARP) and the California Association for Concerned Senior Citizens (CACSC) to stop selling insurance in that state. These organizations play on the similarity of their names to those of senior organizations such as the American Association of Retired Persons to sell insurance to seniors.

Sales Practices To Watch Out For

There are a number of sales practices that older health consumers should watch out for when shopping for supplemental health insurance. For example, an insurance agent named William John McKernan was arrested in Jupiter, Florida, in February of 1989 for selling older health-care consumers policies that they couldn't use. By his own account he made $60,000 in 1988 selling useless policies to seniors. One Canadian woman lost more than a thousand dollars on a Medicare supplemental policy that she could not use because she was not covered by Medicare. The victim is an intelligent, savvy woman, not one to be easily fooled. However, she was taken in by the agent because she thought the policy would cover her for foreign travel. It could happen to anyone. Here are insurance sales practices that older consumers should watch out for. They include:

Impersonating a Government Official. The agent says he or she is from Medicare or another government agency.

"Rolling Over." The individual is persuaded to cancel policies and buy new ones, giving the agent a commission.

Duplication. The individual is persuaded to buy policies that duplicate existing coverage.

Theft. The agent persuades the individual to make the check out to him or her or to pay cash. The agent keeps the money and a policy is never written.

Switching. The agent sells the individual one policy and switches it for another when it comes time for the individual to sign, or the agent tells the individual that the total cost of the policy is higher than the receipt the client actually receives.

Clean Sheeting. The agent fails to report preexisting conditions so that the company refuses to pay when claims are filed, or he or she forges the individual's signature on a new policy.

Scare Tactics. The agent scares the individual into buying coverage *now* with comments like, "This policy won't be available next week."

Health Maintenance Organizations

Loosely defined, health maintenance organizations (HMOs) combine aspects of health insurance and fee-for-service physician care in that they both provide and finance health care. In an HMO the patient pays a monthly or annual premium that is usually less than the cost of insurance. In exchange for the fee patients get the security that they will not be charged substantial additional costs for medical care. *In any Medicare HMO patients do not pay the Medicare deductibles.* Although HMOs are considered supplemental Medicare plans, they are not subject to the Baucus Amendment. (See page 89.)

HMOs have their roots in the development of the Western Clinic in Tacoma, Washington, in 1906, when lumbermen and mill owners organized their own prepaid group plan with two physicians, James Yocum and Thomas Curran. The cost was 50 cents a month. HMOs began to spring up during the Depression in spite of objections from legislators and physicians that prepaid plans would stifle free enterprise and downgrade quality. The HMOs of today evolved from models started in the 1930s through the 1950s by industrialist Henry Kaiser, the Teamsters in St. Louis, and the United Auto Workers in Detroit, among others. Notably, Kaiser's prepaid plan would become the patriarch of group plans, the Kaiser-Permanente. Finally, in 1973, Congress passed the Health Maintenance Organization Act, with the goal of standardizing and developing HMOs. The act also designated funding for research into HMO delivery systems. Requirements for federal qualifications under the act are

A basic benefit package

Open enrollment annually

Consumer representation on the board of directors

Coverage based on community rating rather than on experience rating

While HMOs became a 1970s health-care phenomenon for the working-age population and their families, they are a relatively new option for seniors. Until recently HMOs had difficulty getting reimbursed for services to Medicare recipients. However, due to recent changes in government rules, by 1987 there were 1.1 million Medicare beneficiaries in about 150 Medicare HMOs representing 3.5 percent of the Medicare population. Another 580,000 were in similar group arrangements. (For a list of Medicare HMOs, see Table 6.1.)

Confusing matters, Medicare calls some HMOs Competitive Medical Plans (CMPs). CMP refers to plans with a particular kind of government contract, called a risk contract. The majority of Medicare HMOs have risk contracts with lock-in features, which means that neither Medicare nor the HMO will pay anything if the HMO Medicare member goes to a doctor or other

Table 6.1   Medicare-Approved HMOs by Region

Medicare HMOs have received approval from the Health Care Financing Administration (HCFA) to provide services to Medicare beneficiaries. The following is a list of Medicare-approved HMOs by HCFA-designated region.

CITY/TOWN	PLAN NAME
BOSTON REGION	
Amherst	Kaiser
Boston	Harvard Community Health Plan
Boston	Lahey Clinic
Braintree	Med East Community Health Plan
Cambridge	Bay State Health Care
Chicopee	Med West Community Health Plan
Hartford	Kaiser Foundation Health Plan
Norwalk	Prucare Plus
Providence	Rhode Island Group Health Association
Trumbull	Physicians Health Service
Warwick	Ocean State Physician Health Plan
Washua	Matt Thorn Health Plan
Wellesley	Multigroup Health Plan
Woodridge	Health Care Inc.
Worcester	Fallow Community Health Plan
NEW YORK REGION	
Albany	Capital Area
Buffalo	Health Care Plan of Buffalo
District of Columbia	Network Health Plan Corp.
Great Neck	Total Health
Greater New York City	Health Insurance Plan of New York
Greater New York City	United States Health Care Inc.
Hauppauge	Prucare
Iselin	Healthways
Medford	Health Care Plan/Health Insurance Plan
Paramus	Health Insurance Plan of New Jersey
Parsippany	Prucare Plus
Pittsburgh	Maxicare/Health American
Poughkeepsie	Health Shield
Rochester	Blue Choice
Rochester	Genesee Valley
Rochester	Preferred Care Health Plan
Short Hills	Foundation Health Plan
Somerset	Rutgers Community Health Plan
Vineland	Omnicare
Westchester County	Kaiser Foundation Health Plan
PHILADELPHIA REGION	
Baltimore	Care First
Baltimore	Johns Hopkins Health Plan
Baltimore Metro	Kaiser Mid Atlantic
Blue Bell	HMO Pennsylvania
District of Columbia Metro	Maryland-Individual Practassociation
Philadelphia	Maxicare Philadelphia
Philadelphia	Prucare Plus
Richmond	Prucare Plus

Table 6.1   (continued)

CITY/TOWN	PLAN NAME

PHILADELPHIA REGION

| Riverdale | Health Plus |
| Washington | Prudential Senior Plus |

ATLANTA REGION

Atlanta	Health 1st, Inc.
Atlanta	Kaiser-Georgia
Atlanta	Prucare Plus
Charlotte	Prucare Plus
Daytona Beach	Florida Health Care Plan
Fort Lauderdale	Prucare Plus
Jackson	Prucare Plus
Louisville	Humana Health Plan
Memphis	Prudential Medicare Plus
Miami	AV-Med Health Plan
Miami	CAC–Comprehensive America Care
Miami	Health Options of Southern Florida
Miami	Heritage
Miami	Humana Medical Plan
Nashville	Prudential Medicare Plus
Orlando	Prucare Plus
Raleigh	Kaiser of North Carolina
Tallahassee	Capital Health Plan
Tampa	Prucare Plus

CHICAGO REGION

Bellaire	Bellaire
Bloomington	Share
Chicago	Anchor
Chicago	Health Chicago
Chicago	Michael Reese Health Plan
Chicago	Share Illinois
Cleveland	Kaiser-Akron
Cleveland	Kaiser-Ohio
Des Plaines	Prucare
Detroit	Health Alliance
Duluth	HMO Minnesota/Blue Plus
Elm Grove	Foundation Health Plan Coop
Flint	Health Plus
Indianapolis	Metro Health
Indianapolis	Prucare Plus
Kalamazoo	Physician Health Plan of Michigan
Lansing	Health Central
Marion	Health Ohio
Metro and South East	HMO Minnesota/Blue Plus
Minneapolis	Group Health Inc.
Minneapolis	Medcenters Health Plan
Minnetonka	Physician Health Plan of Minnesota
Northeast	HMO Minnesota/Blue Plus
St. Paul	HMO Midwest
St. Paul	North Western National Life Health Network

Table 6.1   (continued)

CITY/TOWN	PLAN NAME
DALLAS REGION	
Albuquerque	Foundation Health Plan New Mexico
Albuquerque	Lovelace Health Plan
Austin	Prudential Classic Health Plan
Corpus Christi	Humana
Dallas	Prucare HMO
Dallas	Sanus Health Plan of Dallas
Dallas, Fort Worth	Kaiser of Texas
Houston	Prucare-Houston
Houston	Sanus Health Plan of Houston
Little Rock	Prucare Plus
Oklahoma City	Prudential Senior Plus
San Antonio	Humana Health Plan of Texas
San Antonio	Pacificare of Texas
San Antonio	Prudential Classic Health Plan
Tulsa	Prucare of Tulsa
Tulsa	Prucare Plus
KANSAS CITY REGION	
Davenport	Heritage National Health Plan
Des Moines	Share Iowa
Kansas City	Prucare Plus
Lincoln	Maxicare/Health AN Nebraska
Omaha	Share Nebraska
Rugby	Heart of America
St. Louis	Sanus Health Plan
South Central State	HMO Kansas South Central
Wichita	Equicor
Wichita	HMO Kansas Wichita
DENVER REGION	
Alamosa	HMO Health Plans
Canon City	Qual-Med, Upper Arkansas Valley
Colorado Springs	Peak Health Plan Ltd.
Colorado Springs	Qual-Med, Colorado Springs
Denver	Comprecare, Inc.
Denver	HMO Colorado
Denver	Kaiser Colorado
Denver	Prucare Plus
Denver Area	Qual-Med, Denver Area
Grand Junction	Rocky Mountain
Pueblo	Qual-Med, Pueblo Area
SAN FRANCISCO REGION	
Bakersfield	Kaiser Foundation Health Plan
Fount Valley	Foundation Health Plan
Honolulu	Hawaiian Medical Service Assoc.
Honolulu	Kaiser Foundation
Inglewood	United Health Plan (Watts)
Las Vegas	Health Plan of Nevada/South
Lihue	Island Care
Martinez	Contra Costa
Orange County	Pacificare (Secure Horizon)

Table 6.1   (continued)

CITY/TOWN	PLAN NAME
SAN FRANCISCO REGION	
Pasadena	Kaiser/Southern
Phoenix	Cigna Arizona
Phoenix	Foundation Health Plan Arizona
Phoenix	Humana Health Plan of Arizona
Reno	Health Plan of Nevada
Sacramento	Health Care
San Bernardino	Inland Health Plan
San Bernardino	Intervalley Health Plan
San Diego	Prucare Plus
San Francisco	Children's Hospital
San Francisco	French Hospital
San Francisco	Prucare Plus
South Bay Area	Bay Pacific
SEATTLE REGION	
Portland	Good Health Plan of Oregon
Portland	HMO of Oregon
Portland	Kaiser–North West
Portland	Physician Association of Clackamus County
Portland	Secure Horizons
Seattle	Group Health of Puget Sound
Seattle	Network Health Plan
Spokane	Group Health North West

provider outside the HMO. The HMO member would have to pay the entire bill. Exceptions include emergency cases and authorized referrals when an HMO does not provide a specific service. In addition, HMOs with risk contracts must use any savings to increase benefits or to lower any premiums they may charge. HMOs may also have another kind of contract with Medicare, called a cost contract.

Eligibility for a Medicare HMO

To be eligible for a Medicare HMO, seniors must be enrolled in Medicare's Part B and continue to pay the Part B premium. Also they must either have Part A of Medicare or pay a higher monthly premium to the HMO. Patients must also live in the HMO's geographical area for at least nine months of the year.

Medicare recipients cannot be denied enrollment to an HMO because of advanced age, or for any preexisting medical condition no matter how severe, with the exception of end-stage kidney failure. Medicare HMOs are required to have at least one 30-day open-enrollment period every year when individuals may sign up.

HMOs provide all services that Medicare recipients are entitled to, as well as some additional ones. Many HMOs cover inpatient hospitalization costs in full, including the deductible. Other services may include immunizations, prescription drugs at reduced cost, and routine eye care, for example. A survey conducted in 1987 found that Medicare HMOs are more flexible in providing nonmedically related home health services than traditional Medicare. A third of HMOs offer supplemental home health services that are not covered by Medicare.

The costs and benefits of HMOs vary from plan to plan. According to law, HMOs can charge beneficiaries a monthly fee that is equivalent to the coinsurance and deductible amounts that they would have paid under traditional Medicare.

Here are ten points for seniors to consider when shopping for HMOs.

1. HMO subscribers have fewer out-of-pocket expenses. All HMO physicians "accept assignment" from Medicare as payment in full. An office call is either free or for a small cost. Hospitalization is paid for completely. Subscribers pay no Medicare deductibles.

2. The HMO handles the paperwork. Subscribers don't have to file any claims.

3. Selection of physicians and hospitals is limited to those contracting with the HMO. Subscribers choose the doctor from a list provided by the HMO and can't see specialists without approval from the "primary care physician" (internist or family doctor).

4. In some cases, care may be given by nurse practitioners or others under the supervision of the doctor, but not directly by the doctor.

5. Subscribers who are unhappy with their HMO doctor can choose another HMO doctor, and those dissatisfied with an HMO may leave it. Subscribers may not be able to join another HMO right away, because the "open enrollment" period could be over. However, seniors would still have their Medicare coverage if they left the HMO.

6. All health-care services must be received through the HMO. Neither the HMO nor Medicare will pay for services received elsewhere (such as from a nonparticipating doctor). One exception: when the HMO refers subscribers elsewhere for a needed service that the HMO cannot provide. The other exception is emergency care. The HMO defines "emergency" very strictly. Also, follow-up care for the emergency must be obtained through the HMO in the subscriber's local area. Thus, HMOs might not meet the health-care needs of individuals who travel frequently. Check individual programs carefully—some large HMOs offer "reciprocity," which allows access to their services in other cities and states.

7. Monthly premium rates are guaranteed for one year only. They could go up next year.

8. Medicare HMO plans are meant to be inclusive health-care plans that replace the need for supplemental insurance, or medigap policies. But subscribers who leave an HMO and then reapply for supplemental insurance could have difficulty or added expense if they have a serious preexisting medical condition.

9. The HMO doesn't cover every possible health problem. Therefore, it is important to compare benefit levels among plans.

10. If the HMO goes out of business, subscribers are fully covered through the benefit year. If the HMO decides to drop its Medicare plan, it must give subscribers 60 days' advance written notice.

Preferred Provider Organizations

Preferred Provider Organizations (PPOs) are a variation on both the HMO and fee-for-service plans in which a group-insurance purchaser agrees to send participants to particular hospitals, doctors, or organizations in exchange for a "volume discount." PPOs keep prices down for health consumers and provide a steady flow of clients for health providers. Early in 1989 five demonstration projects were selected to test the possibility of offering Medicare beneficiaries the option of selecting physicians through a PPO. Beneficiaries who live near any of these project sites can reduce out-of-pocket costs through using their services: Blue Cross/Blue Shield, Phoenix, Arizona; Healthlink, St. Louis, Missouri; Caremark, Portland, Oregon; Family Health Plan, Minneapolis, Minnesota; and Capp Care, Fountain Valley, California.

Medicaid Benefits

Medicaid is an assistance program that pays for medical care for people who have limited income and cannot afford insurance. Medicaid was established by Congress along with Medicare in 1965 as an amendment to the Social Security Act. Medicaid and Medicare, while often confused, differ greatly. (See Table 6.2.) For example, Medicare has uniform standards; within certain guidelines, Medicaid leaves standards up to the states. While Medicare has a set rate for fees from physicians, they are allowed to charge more; Medicaid also has a set rate, but physicians are not allowed to charge more.

Table 6.2   A Comparison of Medicare and Medicaid

MEDICARE	MEDICAID
What Are Medicare and Medicaid?	
Insurance Program	Assistance Program
Run by Federal Government	Run by States
Services Are Same throughout the United States	Programs Vary by State
Does Not Discriminate	Does Not Discriminate
Eligibility	
Social Security and Railroad Retirement Recipients	Very Low Income Requirements
Working Together	
10% of People with Medicare Also Have Medicaid	Some Medicaid Recipients Also Have Medicare
Medicare Pays Part, Not All	Medicaid Can Pay What Medicare Does Not
Medicare Part B Charges a Premium	Medicaid Pays the Medicare Premium

Table 6.2   (continued)

MEDICARE	MEDICAID
Services	
Has Two Parts	Programs Vary by State
Covers Only Skilled Care	Covers Long-Term Care
Availability	
Both Available in All States, the District of Columbia, Guam, Puerto Rico, and the Virgin Islands	
Numbers Covered	
Covers About 33 Million	Covers About 23 Million
91% Are Elderly	14% Are Elderly
Financing	
Workers, Their Employers, the Federal Government, and Beneficiaries Pay	Federal and State Pay
Applying	
Medicare Card Automatically Sent to Beneficiaries or Apply at Social Security Office	Apply at Welfare Office
Federal Responsibility	
HCFA Responsible for Administration	HCFA Responsible for Federal Aspects of the Program

Medicaid is financed by federal and state governments. In 1987, 3.3 million persons age 65 and older received $16.1 billion in Medicaid vendor payments. In many states, recipients of Supplemental Security Income automatically qualify for Medicaid. States design their own Medicaid program within federal guidelines, and eligibility and benefits vary accordingly. New York, for instance, spent $2.9 billion on 353,061 elderly Medicaid recipients in 1987, while California spent $743 million on 539,160 elderly residents. Thirty-eight states provide Medicaid assistance to individuals who have large medical bills that would put their income below a certain level. These individuals are referred to as "medically needy." In 1987 the states that did not have "medically needy" programs were Delaware, Alabama, Mississippi, Indiana, Ohio, New Mexico, Missouri, South Dakota, Wyoming, Nevada, Alaska, and Hawaii.

Ten percent of the elderly were eligible for both Medicare and Medicaid in 1984, the latest year for which data are available.

Medicare recipients who cannot afford supplemental insurance or low-income individuals not eligible for Medicare should investigate the possibility of receiving help from Medicaid. When individuals are eligible for both Medicare and Medicaid, Medicaid often pays for Medicare's premiums, deductibles, and coinsurance amounts. Older adults with Medicaid do not need supplemental health insurance. Unfortunately, however, a recent survey by the American Association of Retired Persons (AARP) found that as many as half of all older Medicaid beneficiaries unnecessarily purchase medigap coverage. AARP estimates that 1.8 million older Medicaid recipients pay as much as $705 a year for insurance that they do not need.

To be eligible for Medicaid an individual must meet certain income and asset tests. The following are additional rules for Medicaid eligibility:

The applicant must be 65 or older, or blind or disabled, or be a parent of a minor child.

The applicant must be a U.S. citizen or a legal alien. However, aliens granted amnesty in the current amnesty program are ineligible for five years.

The applicant must be a resident of the state in which he or she is applying.

Medicaid covers the following services to some extent in all states:

Inpatient hospital care

Outpatient services

Other laboratory and X-ray services

Skilled-nursing-facility services

Home health care services

Rural health-clinic services

In addition, most states cover:

Dental care

Prescribed drugs

Eyeglasses

Clinic services

Intermediate-care services

Usually a state's department of social services is the place to apply for Medicaid. A decision on an application may take up to three months. Applicants need the following when they apply: proof of age, citizenship, and residency; Social Security number; income and resource records; and proof of medical expenses.

Financial Assistance for Low-Income Medicare Beneficiaries

The Medicare Catastrophic Coverage Act of 1988, which was repealed in 1989, provided some assistance for paying for the Medicare premium and at least some of the deductibles and copayments for low-income individuals. The program is often referred to as the "Medicaid buy in." Fortunately, the "buy in" was *not* repealed but was retained because of its importance to low-income Americans. To be eligible, participants must meet some income and resource requirements and must not otherwise be eligible for Medicaid. The Congressional Committee on Ways and Means estimates that 8 percent of Medicare enrollees may benefit from the buy in. The maximum income level for qualification may vary by state, but generally annual income must fall below the national poverty level ($5,770 for one person or $7,730 for a family of two in January 1989). The date of availability will vary by state. As of this writing many states have not yet instituted their programs. State and local welfare offices and social-service or public-health offices will provide information about the program.

Veterans' Benefits

Older health consumers who are eligible for veterans' benefits may receive more comprehensive coverage than they would under Medicare. For example, in addition to hospitalization, veterans with service-related disabilities may qualify for treatment in a Department of Veterans Affairs (VA) or private nursing home if needed.

Because of great demand on the Department of Veterans Affairs system, there is a hierarchy for which veterans receive services first. Veterans who are farthest down on the priority list will be considered last. Here is the hierarchy for hospitalization:

1. Veterans needing hospitalization due to injury or disease incurred or aggravated in the line of duty in active service.

2. Veterans who were discharged or retired because of disabilities incurred or aggravated in the line of duty and who are receiving or did receive compensation for those disabilities, but who need treatment for another ailment not connected with the service.

3. Certain veterans who do not meet the criteria above but apply for treatment of non-service-connected disabilities. All veterans who are age 65 or older are in these categories. They are admitted to the hospital if beds are available. Unfortunately, because of the large number of veterans in this age group, only those in less-populated areas will be admitted.

Since 1986 the VA has been charging copayments to veterans whose income is over a certain level and who have non-service-connected conditions for treatment in a VA hospital or medical facility, or for other VA authorized treatment.

Admission to VA nursing homes follows essentially the same pattern as that for hospitals. Veterans with service-related disabilities receive priority. Local VA offices handle applications for veterans' benefits. Organizations such as the Veterans of Foreign Wars and the American Legion also provide assistance.

A Medicare beneficiary who is also eligible for VA benefits can choose to receive treatment under either program. Medicare will not pay for services furnished by VA hospitals and VA medical facilities, except for certain emergency hospital services. Also, Medicare will not pay for services that the VA is authorized to pay. In some cases Medicare will reimburse beneficiaries for copayments charged to them by the VA.

Catastrophic or Major Medical Insurance

Catastrophic or major medical policies help cover the costs of serious injury or illness, including some services not covered by Medicare. These policies are not Medicare supplemental policies and may not cover Medicare's deductibles and copayments. These policies are not generally a good buy for Medicare beneficiaries.

Indemnity and Other Limited Policies

There are several types of limited policies that may be advertised by celebrities and may sound like wise choices. *However, they are not designed to fill in Medicare's gaps and generally are not good buys for older persons.*

Hospital Indemnity Policies

Indemnity policies pay a fixed amount each day, week, or month while patients are in the hospital. They pay benefits regardless of whether the subscriber has other hospital coverage. However, benefits cannot be collected unless the patient is hospitalized. Hospital indemnity policies are not wise choices for filling in Medicare's gaps.

Accident-Only Policies

Accident-only policies provide coverage for death, dismemberment, or hospital and medical care due to an accident. They are not designed to pay routine health-care costs.

Dread-Disease Policies

Dread-disease policies insure individuals for specific diseases such as cancer. These policies are sometimes referred to as specified-disease policies. They pay in so few situations that they are banned for sale in a number of states. They are not good options for filling in Medicare's gaps.

Travel-accident and intensive-care policies are also often marketed to the elderly. These are very limited in scope and do not fill in the gaps left by Medicare.

Insurance Options Prior to Becoming a Medicare Recipient

Health-care consumers who are between retirement and age 65 (when eligibility for Medicare begins) have two major options. In most cases, the first option is preferable:

Continuing group insurance. In 1986 three-quarters of health-plan participants in medium-size and large firms were entitled to health coverage between retirement and age 65. In some cases the employer pays part of the cost.

Purchasing individual insurance and switching to a supplemental policy at age 65. This is sometimes the only choice. Individual policies are expensive. However, it is dangerous to go without any kind of health-insurance protection.

Chapter 7

Paying for Long-Term Care

- Long-term care is that combination of services that provides health-related and supportive services to mildly to severely incapacitated individuals who require care for a long period of time. Long-term-care services may be delivered at home or in a nursing home.
- About 70 percent of older persons who receive long-term-care services at home pay the bills out of their own pockets.
- About half of the costs of the nation's nursing-home bill is paid for by residents and their families.
- Medicare does not pay for long-term care in a nursing home or at home. Medicare supplemental policies also do not pay for long-term care.
- In order for Medicaid to cover nursing-home costs, residents must meet Medicaid's low-income guidelines and must be medically in need of the service.
- Four out of five persons who need long-term care live in the community, not in nursing homes.

Introduction

Ideally, long-term-care services give physically limited individuals the gifts of independence and quality of life. Long-term care

111

can be defined as the wide range of medical and support services provided to persons who have lost some or all capacity to function on their own. The factor that distinguishes it from other services, such as skilled-nursing care, is that the person receiving the service will require help for a long period of time, usually as long as he or she lives. While many think of long-term care as nursing-home care, the truth is that the vast majority of long-term-care services are provided in the comforts of home, not in an institution. And there are increasing numbers of high-quality alternative community services that, when coordinated, make long-term care at home possible.

This chapter looks at who needs long-term care, in-home and nursing-home care services, long-term-care insurance, and other options for financing long-term care.

The Need for Long-Term Care

Older adults are in need of long-term care if, due to a health problem, they have difficulty performing necessary tasks ranging from shopping to bathing. Individuals may require long-term care as the result of an acute illness such as stroke or as the result of a chronic problem such as arthritis. There is great diversity in the types and degrees of services required by those in need of long-term care. For example, Mrs. Smith, who has arthritis, requires stable, low-intensity services, while her neighbor, Mrs. Jones, receives dialysis treatments at home. Both Mrs. Smith and Mrs. Jones are making use of long-term-care services.

Long-term-care needs also change over time. Over a 20-year period, a woman with severe arthritis may go from needing minimal help around the house to 24-hour care, for instance. And during that period of time if she falls and breaks a hip, she may need short-term rehabilitative care and then recover and go back to requiring less-intensive but steady care.

The common assumption that most elderly receive long-term care in nursing homes is, fortunately, a myth. An estimated four out of five elderly who need long-term care live in the community. Only one in five lives in a nursing home.

Help in the Home

In 1984, the latest year for which data are available, there were 5.3 million elderly persons in need of long-term care at home. Almost 3 million of these required extensive services due to severe disability. According to the Health Industry Manufacturers Association, in 1990 Americans will spend $11.2 billion on home health care services and $4.8 billion on related products.

Who Pays for Care at Home

The $14-billion home health care industry does not necessarily provide care that is less expensive than nursing-home care, but for many older adults it means the difference between receiving services in the comfortable, familiar environment of home rather than the institutional environment of a nursing home. About 70 percent of all older people who use home-care services pay the bill out of their own pockets, but most care is provided by family and friends with no direct expense attached. Eighty-four percent of all care givers for disabled elderly males living outside of institutions are relatives. This figure is 79 percent for elderly women.

The most common method of payment for long-term care at home is a fee paid by the service recipient or family members. Home care is estimated to cost an average of $40 a day, but it can run as high as $60,000 a year for full-time care. There is no one program or central federal source that pays for long-term care. There are four major federal programs that sometimes will pay for such care, however. They are Medicaid, Older Americans Act programs (through Area Agencies on Aging), Social Service Block Grants, and Medicare. Most states also provide some services through general revenues, and a limited number of private health-insurance policies, Department of Veterans Affairs programs, health maintenance organizations, and social-service organizations will help with long-term-care costs. In addition, some long-term-care insurance policies also sometimes provide help for those older health consumers who can afford the premiums.

The following is a brief description of these general sources of long-term-care funding. Long-term-care insurance's role in funding home health care is described separately beginning on page 133.

Medicaid

Medicaid is by far the dominant federal program for funding long-term care at home. To receive home health care through Medicaid an older person must meet state guidelines for Medicaid, and then the state Medicaid program must determine that the individual needs the service. Availability of home health care through Medicaid varies greatly by state. For example, in 1986 approximately half of all Medicaid users of home health care lived in New York State. And, including New York, three-quarters of users resided in just eight states. For information on becoming eligible for Medicaid, see page 104.

Older Americans Act Programs

Older Americans Act programs (OAA) are important vehicles of long-term care, even though their overall share of total costs is relatively small. The Older Americans Act was passed in 1965 as part of President Johnson's Great Society program after the 1961 White House Conference brought attention to the need for community services to older Americans. The act has been amended a number of times since then, including a lowering of the target population for services from age 65 to 60. However, the act's primary goal has remained essentially the same: to provide a wide array of social and community services to those older persons in the greatest economic and social need in order to foster maximum independence. A sampling of some of the services supported by the act includes information and referral services, home-care services, meal programs, senior centers, and nursing-home ombudsman services.

In 1988 Congress appropriated $1.2 billion for Older Americans Act programs, which is insignificant by federal budget standards. The Older Americans Act has several titles supporting important community programs. Title III is the most significant part of the act, delineating the types of services that should be available at the local level. In addition, the act designates a state agency with responsibility for services for the aging. These agencies, called State Units on Aging (SUAs), are identified by the governor as responsible for overseeing aging services. SUAs may be independent departments or commissions on aging or part of the state's human-services agency. In 28 states SUAs are part of a human-services department, and in another 21 states the office is independent. SUAs, in turn, commonly distribute funds to Area Agencies on Aging (AAAs), which are smaller agencies throughout a state, although a few states have only one central agency. There are more than 600 AAAs throughout the country serving more than 2 million elderly. AAAs fund local services to older adults on a non-means-tested basis. However, waiting lists are long. Information on local Older Americans Act programs is available through state units on aging listed in Chapter 10.

Social Service Block Grants

The Social Service Block Grant (SSBG) program is the major source of federal funding for social-service programs in the states. The program is designed to assist families and individuals in maintaining self-sufficiency and independence. In 1987 Congress allotted $2.7 billion to the states for SSBG programs, all of which must be spent on social-service programs. However, it is not known how much of this amount goes for programs serving older adults. SSBG programs serve people of all ages, and each state determines how SSBG funds will be spent. In 1986 all 50 states, the District of Columbia, and the four eligible territories all spent SSBG funds on home-based services.

Other block-grant programs also make funds available to states that may be used for long-term care, including the Alcohol/Drug Abuse and Mental Health Block Grants, Community Development Block Grants, and Energy Assistance Block Grants. Information on local SSBG and related block-grant programs is available through relevant state units on aging listed in Chapter 10 and community social-service agencies.

Medicare

Medicare does not contribute toward long-term care except for limited respite and skilled-nursing care. Payments for home health care equal only 4 percent of total Medicare outlays. *An important rule of thumb for Medicare beneficiaries: never contract for home health care services under the assumption that Medicare or another agency is going to pay for it.*

Other Sources of Funding for Care at Home

A very small number of supplemental health-insurance policies will pay part of the costs of long-term care under limited circumstances. Policyholders should check to see whether their plan offers such coverage. In addition, some older veterans are eligible for Department of Veterans Affairs home health benefits, and a growing number of health maintenance organizations offer home health services. But overall these sources are very limited. Finally, the most common method of payment for long-term care is a fee paid by the service recipient or family members.

Noninstitutional Health and Related Services

The following noninstitutional health and related services are available in most communities. The needs for these services almost always overlap and, to be effective, they should be personalized. In addition, the appropriate mix of services should be adjusted as needs change over time. Programs that are usually free are marked with a star (★). When Medicare or other federal programs pay for a service, it is indicated.

Location, Coordination, and Counseling Services

These services provide the means to locate and personalize in-home or community programs:

INFORMATION AND REFERRAL SERVICES (I&R) are the link between older persons and their families, who are far too often unaware of what is available to them and to community services. I&R services began in the 1960s when social programs began to increase, creating a demand for information on what services were available and how to gain access to them. In 1973 amendments to the Older Americans Act made information and referral services for the elderly a priority.

I&R services maintain continuously updated file systems that list health services, community organizations, service providers, and business resources in the area. Information and referral workers also do social work and counseling, and they identify gaps in services. Anonymity is guaranteed, and the service may be provided by telephone or through outreach.

The types of questions that information and referral services receive generally involve access to benefits such as SSI or Medicaid; home health care and related services; nursing-home care; transportation; employment counseling; legal aid; and health problems and care. Many questions come from family members rather than older persons themselves. The major sources for information and referral services for older persons are local aging offices. In 1988 Area Agencies on Aging handled approximately 11 million telephone information and referral phone calls. *Medicare and Medicaid do not pay for information and referral services.*

CASE MANAGERS coordinate services across the board, from home health care to transportation to physical therapy. Many also provide counseling. Case managers are particularly important because of their role of personalizing and coordinating long-term-care services. They are situated in aging, social-service, and home-care offices. *Medicare does not pay for case management. However, some state Medicaid programs will.*

Private case managers offer their services to older persons and their families for a fee. They are sometimes referred to as private geriatric-care managers. *Their services are expensive, often ranging from $50 to $75 an hour, but a good case manager can save a client hundreds of dollars and provide ease of mind to relatives.* Private case managers arrange for such services as housing, home health care, transportation, and nursing home placement. Most are also on 24-hour call. Often their clients are the children of aging parents who live far away from their parents and need someone to coordinate care for their parent.

Because there is potential for abuse in this area, it is important to use only the services of case managers who are licensed by the state. Often hospital discharge workers and information and referral workers in aging offices are good sources of information for trustworthy private case managers. Two other good sources of information are Aging Network Services and the National Association of Private Geriatric Care Managers.

Home-Care Services

These services encompass a wide range of supportive services for individuals who are homebound. They are often credited with allowing people to remain at home and out of nursing homes. The following services are available in most communities.

Home-care services offer a variety of programs, from sophisticated therapies (health care) to preparing meals (homemaking). Home-care agencies may provide their services through hospitals, nursing homes, public-health agencies, social-service agencies, or other organizations. There are three descending levels of intensity of services for home care:

1. SKILLED NURSING is often referred to as home health care and is care for those with acute problems, such as cardiac seizure or a terminal illness requiring intravenous feeding. Skilled nursing is generally not considered a long-term-care program because its purpose is to take care of acute problems. Skilled nursing is defined as that provided by a licensed professional nurse or therapist, whereas unskilled care is provided by an aide, companion, attendant, or personal-care worker. *Skilled nursing is the most likely to qualify for Medicare coverage. This type of care must be ordered by a physician in order to be eligible for Medicare. Many group-insurance policies now have provisions for skilled care.*

The following two types of service are provided by in-home service workers, usually called homemaker–home health aides, or by an aide, companion, attendant, or personal-care worker. The services they perform may range from cleaning and cooking to doing the laundry and shampooing the patient's hair.

2. PERSONAL OR INTERMEDIATE SERVICES are for individuals whose acute or chronic conditions have stabilized and whose main need is for help in activities such as bathing, meal preparation, taking medicines, and physical therapy.

3. HOMEMAKER, CHORE, OR BASIC SERVICES are for individuals who do not require medical care but need help with meal preparation and housekeeping. *The latter two services are often referred to as home care, and Medicare covers them only when the recipient also is in need of skilled care and only for as long as skilled care is required. Medicaid covers these services in some states.*

Supplemental insurance policies rarely pay for personal or homemaker services.

Home-care agencies have flourished over the past decade, and there are now more than 10,000 home-care agencies. Unfortunately, however, because of lack of funding, the demand for home care is greater than the supply. Home-care agencies may be privately run, for-profit, or nonprofit. Many are hospital connected; more than 70 percent of all hospitals now have home-care programs. Agencies that provide Medicare-reimbursed services must be certified, but generally the home-care network is unregulated. The National Homecaring Council (NHC) in New York accredits homemaker/home health aide services. Older persons may want to contact the council to see which agencies in a particular area are certified by NHC.

The quality and cost of home-care services vary tremendously. Sources for locating home-care services include friends who have had personal experience with agencies, local aging organizations, discharge workers, and local social-service agencies. Consumers should avoid locating agencies through the Yellow Pages or advertisements and letting their staff into their homes without first getting recommendations from friends and family, or from professional sources such as local aging organizations or hospital discharge workers.

Home-care services are billed by the hour or visit. Costs vary greatly by region and by the degree of skilled care required. At the highest end of the scale, for instance, are occupational or speech therapists; next in line are nurses; and aides are the least expensive source of care in the home.

A variety of agencies provide in-home services. The type of agency is usually defined by the type of service that is provided and by whether funding is received through a public or a private source. Generally home health agencies are community based, hospital based, public, nonprofit, or for-profit.

Other In-Home Services

In addition to home health care, most communities also have an extensive network of in-home services that enable older persons to remain in their homes. A number of these services overlap with the in-home services described above and may be provided by the same aide or agency that also provides an older client with home health care. The best resource for these services is local aging organizations.

CHORE SERVICES offer help in and around the house, including minor repairs, heavy housecleaning, and yard work. *These services are not covered by Medicare. However, some states and some Older Americans Act programs will pay for chore services.*

HOME-DELIVERED MEALS, often referred to as meals-on-wheels, are prepared meals delivered to individuals in their homes. The concept of home-delivered meals was begun in England following World War II. The first program in the United States started in Philadelphia in 1955. Meals-on-wheels programs are usually staffed by volunteers who deliver the meals, frequently working in pairs and providing friendly visiting for the recipients as well as a nutritious meal. Sometimes special diets are available. *Usually there is a fixed fee or a sliding scale.*

Many meal programs are funded through the Older Americans Act, and frequently local organizations also contribute. The goal of OAA-sponsored programs is to provide one to two meals a day for five days a week. Unfortunately, waiting lists are generally long. To qualify for OAA-sponsored home-delivered meals, individuals must be age 60 or older. Such programs serve only those who are designated as homebound by specific medical criteria. *Food stamps may be used for home-delivered meals, and an aide or relative can apply for them for the recipient.*

★ FRIENDLY VISITING provides regular companionship to older persons who may be lonely and isolated. Friendly visiting is actually a formalization of an ancient tradition of visiting those in need. Such programs are usually run by volunteers, who do everything from writing letters for older persons to helping them shop. Friendly-visiting programs are generally organized to serve older adults in their homes. However, a number of programs are now also available for older persons in nursing homes. State nursing-home ombudsman offices (in state units on aging) have information about friendly-visiting programs.

★ ESCORT SERVICES accompany older people on health visits or to run errands. In some high-crime communities, escort services are organized by the police for the protection of the older person. Bilingual escorts are often available. Escort services may be located through local aging offices.

★ TELEPHONE REASSURANCE is a community program in which daily telephone calls are made to "check in" with persons living alone. The first program was started in Michigan in the 1960s by Grace McClure, who found an elderly friend on the floor after a stroke. Telephone reassurance programs are run by volunteers. If a volunteer calls the older person's home and no one answers the phone, he or she will seek help quickly, calling the neighbors first and then the police. In rural areas mail carriers often provide a similar service when they check on elderly residents who live on their carrier routes. For many people who are isolated, knowing that someone is going to check in with them on a regular basis eases the fear that they might fall and be unable to move or have a stroke and not be found.

EMERGENCY RESPONSE SYSTEMS (ERSs), often referred to as life-lines, provide contact with immediate help such as police or rescue squads. The advantage of lifelines is that they provide a 24-hour link between the older adult at home and a medical facility. The systems work through a transmitter carried by the user and a receiver connected to the individual's phone. If the user pushes a button on the transmitter, the phone receiver automatically dials an emergency number. Emergency response systems can be set to call for help when the user is unable to do so. They can be set so that they will call for an emergency response if the user has not used the telephone or pushed a designated button for a set period of time.

ERSs may be located through local hospitals, social-service agencies, nursing homes, and sometimes national centers. *There is a charge for most ERS programs, which can be purchased, rented, or leased. Medicare and Medicaid do not cover ERSs. Some insurance companies may cover the service when it is medically indicated.*

HOSPICE SERVICES provide physical, social, and emotional care for the terminally ill and their families. Hospice refers to a philosophy of care based on the concept of death with dignity. The focus is on pain relief, and the dying person is able to remain with family and friends during his or her last days. Hospices believe in serving the whole person and his or her family. Services usually are provided in the individual's home, but residential services are also available.

There are a number of home-care models of hospice services. Local programs may rely on a coalition model, which coordinates services with other agencies, or a single hospice center may provide a comprehensive range of services. Home-care hospices often are affiliated with a hospital. *As discussed in Chapter 2, Medicare now covers hospice services in qualified agencies. However, older persons should be careful when picking a hospice; only one out of five is certified by Medicare.* For more information on hospice services, see page 33.

RESPITE SERVICES provide short-term relief (respite) to families caring for frail, elderly members. Respite services encompass home care and institutional care and can vary from part of a day to several weeks. *Medicare does not presently pay for respite care. (A respite benefit was included in the Medicare Catastrophic Coverage Act, which was repealed late in 1989.) Some state Medicaid programs pay for respite services.*

Services in the Community

Services in the community complement in-home services, providing valuable assistance to older persons and providing contact with friends, neighbors, and others in the community. The following programs are available in most communities. Programs that are generally free are marked with a star (★).

TRANSPORTATION SERVICES help those who don't drive or who can't use public transportation to get around. Communities may receive funding for special transportation programs in a number of ways. The federal government provides funding through the Urban Mass Transit Act for innovative transportation programs such as buses with wheelchair lifts. *Services funded through the Older Americans Act are required to include transportation to and from their programs. Medicaid pays for transportation to and from medical appointments.*

A typical community transportation program offers a service in which a client is taken to a particular location such as a health clinic or shopping center. The program may operate on a demand or regulated schedule. The ride may be in a taxi, a minibus, or a volunteer's car. *Transportation discounts also are generally provided to older persons. In order to qualify for Urban Mass Transit funds, community transportation programs must provide fares reduced by at least 50 percent to the elderly.*

ADULT FOSTER CARE arranges for individuals to live with families. Foster care for adults has been available since the early 1970s. In most foster-care programs no more than four older adults live together in a single home. Foster-care programs are usually run by local human-services departments. *Funds are sometimes available through the Veterans Administration, but the most common method of payment is for the foster home to receive a portion of the older resident's SSI or Social Security checks.* Because foster homes are often not regulated, extreme caution should be used by older adults in choosing foster care without specific guidance from a reputable caseworker, information or referral worker, or related professional.

★ ADULT PROTECTIVE SERVICES (guardianship or conservatorship) provide legal and financial counseling to people unable to manage alone. Legal guardianship should be considered a last resort, reserved for those persons who truly cannot take care of themselves and are in danger of harming themselves or others.

Protective services can be used for the protection of incapacitated older adults with or without their consent. In the latter case a hearing must be held and the older person loses certain rights, while an agency or individual is appointed as legal guardian with the responsibility of managing the older adult's affairs. The loss of rights on the part of the individual is temporary.

The majority of states have passed public-guardianship legislation, each with its own approach to facilitating guardianship for those in danger of harming themselves. In some states the incapacitated older adult can participate in choosing the guardian; in others the individual must accept whomever the court appoints. Generally most states prefer to appoint a relative as guardian, but if a family member is not available, some states identify particular agencies to act as "public guardians." In some states the same agency that provides services to older adults is usually appointed as guardian.

Protective services can provide an opportunity for fraud if the chosen guardian is unscrupulous. This area of the law and of services for the elderly is in flux, and it is hoped that positive changes will be made—both on a federal level and within states—that will strengthen the rights of individuals in need of guardianship.

ADULT DAY CARE originated in Britain in the 1940s when psychiatric hospitals set up outpatient centers. By the 1950s the British had extended the service to geriatric patients, and, in the United States, the Menninger Clinic opened the first geriatric day hospital in 1947.

Adult day care allows older persons who would otherwise be in a nursing home to receive care in the community while remaining at home. Most programs provide services for those who don't need 24-hour care but do need more care than homemaker services offer. Adult-day-care centers provide assistance to clients for parts of each day, customarily five days a week. The clients receive services in a group setting usually providing some combination of the following: limited medical assistance, supervision, social activities, rehabilitative/restorative services, and family counseling. One drawback of adult-day-care centers is that not all can provide transportation to and from the center.

At about a third of the cost of nursing-home placement, adult day care is a cost-effective alternative to a nursing home. *In some states Medicaid will cover the costs of an approved adult-day-care facility for people who are limited physically or mentally. Sometimes Older Americans Act programs will cover adult day care. Most programs, however, rely on fees and contributions.* An excellent resource for locating local adult day care is the National Council on the Aging, which created a National Institute on Adult Daycare in 1979. The institute serves as a focal point for adult day care on a national level.

MULTIPURPOSE SENIOR CENTERS offer a wide spectrum of services nationwide. The first U.S. center organized for older people started in New York in 1943. The centers are one of three major service programs sponsored through the Older Americans Act,

specifically through Title V. Local agencies also often contribute
to the centers, of which there are thousands across the country.
They not only provide a gathering place and recreational activities for older persons but also serve as multipurpose centers. Many run nutrition programs. The senior centers' services
range from square dancing to blood-pressure screening. Often
included are meals, transportation dispatching, information
and referral, health screening, recreation, counseling, employment, legal and protective services, day care, help in fixing up
homes, and educational programs. Many centers also serve
those with special needs such as the deaf or blind. *Generally
senior-center services are free, though voluntary contributions
are encouraged.*

★ NUTRITION SERVICES were formally authorized under the 1973
amendments to the Older Americans Act to provide one hot meal
a day for persons age 60 and over. Nutrition services bring older
adults together for inexpensive, nutritious meals in a social setting such as a senior center or house of worship. Originally
looked down upon as soup lines, the program became respectably
popular in the 1970s. Usually the centers also provide services
and can provide outreach for long-term-care programs.

    *Nutrition centers are not allowed to charge for meals, but vol-
untary contributions are usually requested.* Some centers suggest
the amounts that they prefer for contributions, or envelopes may
be passed so that individuals can anonymously put in what they
can afford to pay. Nutrition programs have become so popular
and funds so tight that in some areas the sites are requiring res-
ervations, notices of cancellations, and a rotating system of
attendance.

LEGAL ASSISTANCE helps older persons and others with problems in
civil matters. Services are provided either by an attorney or
paralegal. Help is frequently furnished for problems with public
benefits such as Medicare and Medicaid and for nursing-home
rights and guardianship or conservatorship.

    Most legal services for the poor elderly are provided through
the Legal Services Corporation (LSC). LSC offices are also excellent sources of information for older adults regarding the benefits available to them. The LSC is an independent corporation

authorized under federal legislation in 1975. Although the Reagan administration made numerous attempts to cut back on LSC programs, the LSC has 306 offices around the country. They provide services to all individuals whose income falls below the federal poverty level, including the elderly.

Legal programs for the elderly are also sometimes supported through the Older Americans Act, block grants, and revenue sharing. Specifically, 1978 amendments to the Older Americans Act require each state agency on aging to make plans for contracting for legal services and to encourage private lawyers to provide legal services to older adults for reduced fees. The American Bar Association also encourages its members to provide pro bono services to the elderly.

Lawyers are not the only professionals who are useful sources of legal help for the elderly. Paralegal programs for the elderly are available in many areas of the country. Paralegals carry out many of the tasks of attorneys, such as preparing briefs and interpreting regulations, but they are not recognized by bar associations. Fortunately for the low-income elderly, they are permitted by federal regulations to handle public-benefits cases. They can be an excellent resource for older adults who wish to appeal Medicaid decisions, for example. The American Association of Retired Persons (AARP) has a growing corps of members who have received paralegal training through the Institute on Law and Aging at George Washington University. AARP's paralegals are required to serve for a while in senior centers, where they aid older adults with legal problems.

Any older adult whose income falls below the federal poverty level is eligible for free or low-cost legal services through the LSC. Two valuable sources of information on the legal rights of older adults are the National Senior Citizens Law Center and the Legal Services Corporation. Area Agencies on Aging offices will have information on the legal-services program available in specific areas.

★ SELF-HELP SUPPORT GROUPS lend peer support for older persons and their families coping with health-related problems such as Alzheimer's or Parkinson's disease. According to Ana Madrzyk, a staff writer for the *Daily Herald* in Chicago, 15 million individuals belong to 750,000 self-help or mutual-support groups for

400 conditions nationwide. One of the best-organized self-help networks serving many elderly people is the Alzheimer's Disease and Related Disorders Association (ADRDA). ADRDA has 200 chapters in all states except Alaska and Mississippi. The association and other support groups offer places where individuals with specific problems and their families can talk out their fears and anxieties about medical problems. A number of them also help members find services and resources.

Many states have a central number that people can call to get information about local self-help programs. For example, The Self-Help Center in Evanston, Illinois, has a 24-hour hotline and a file of 2,000 self-help groups in Illinois. Some of the other states and areas that have self-help clearinghouses are Arizona, California, Connecticut, Iowa, Kansas, Massachusetts, Michigan, Minnesota, Missouri, Nebraska, New Jersey, New York, Oregon, Pennsylvania, Rhode Island, South Carolina, Tennessee, Texas, Vermont, Virginia, Washington, D.C., and Wisconsin.

PHYSICAL FITNESS/EXERCISE PROGRAMS assist older people in staying physically active and healthy. These programs are part of a national campaign to promote exercise as an important health asset for people of all ages. Exercise experts may hold classes in a YMCA or YWCA, senior center, nursing home, hospital, or other facility. Many exercise programs are organized for individuals with specific problems such as arthritis or Parkinson's disease. *Exercise programs for older adults are usually available free of charge or for a nominal charge.* Aging offices and senior centers will have information on local exercise programs.

★ LONG-TERM-CARE OMBUDSMEN work cooperatively with nursing homes and board-and-care homes to improve the quality of life for residents. They serve as patient-rights advocates, investigating and negotiating resolutions to concerns voiced by residents in matters of resident services and care. Additionally, they assist personal-care boarding- and nursing-home staffs to meet the needs and concerns of those who use their facilities, as well as educating the elderly and the community about personal-care boarding homes and nursing homes so that there will be a better understanding and use of the long-term-care system. Further goals of the ombudsman are identifying gaps in services provided and advocating needed improvement in legislation and/ or policies affecting care in these facilities. Those with a complaint about long-term-care programs should contact their state ombudsman through their state unit on aging.

Nursing Homes

Risk Factors for Institutionalization

With advancing age the risk of needing a nursing home increases. According to the 1985 National Nursing Home Survey, the latest data available, 1 percent of persons age 65 to 74 were in nursing homes in that year, compared to 22 percent of those age 85 or older.

Two other major risk factors for entering a nursing home are degree of disability and the lack of a family member or friend to supply help. For example, elderly disabled nursing-home residents are about twice as likely as the disabled elderly living in the community to be limited in the major daily activities of bathing, dressing, toileting, and eating. And 50 percent of all elderly disabled persons living in nursing homes have severe limitations, compared to 15 percent living in the community.

The absence of a spouse or other family member to provide care when it is needed is another critical factor leading to institutionalization. This is borne out by the fact that four out of five care givers to disabled older persons living at home are a friend, spouse, or other family member. (Such care in the home is often referred to as informal care giving.) Only 5 percent of home care is on a paid basis.

Types of Facilities

In 1985 approximately 1.4 million persons age 65 and older were in nursing homes, representing about 5 percent of the elderly. For additional information on nursing homes, see page 26. There are two general types of nursing homes, and they vary by the intensity of the services they provide:

Nursing facilities (NFs) provide around-the-clock supervision and treatment by a registered nurse under the direction of a doctor. NFs serve people who require continual medical services. Older consumers should make sure that any facility they are considering is certified by Medicare and Medicaid. *Medicaid will pay for care in a nursing facility for those who qualify, and Medicare will pay for up to 100 days per benefit period only in those nursing facilities that have been certified as skilled-nursing facilities (SNFs).*

Custodial care, or assisted living, provides group living for those who need supervision but not medical care. Personal assistance in the activities of daily living, such as help in eating, getting out of bed, bathing, dressing, toileting, and supervision in taking medications is provided. This level of care does not require the services of persons with professional medical skills or training. *Medicare and Medicaid do not pay for this type of care.*

The yearly cost of nursing-home care can range from $20,000 to $50,000. As previously mentioned, Medicare does *not* pay for long-term nursing-home care. Moreover, Medicaid pays for nursing-home costs only for those who meet strict low-income qualifications. Long-term-care insurance is also inadequate to cover nursing-home costs. The end result is that, unless a nursing-home resident can qualify for Medicaid (see page 104), the resident and the resident's family will have to pay the entire cost out of pocket.

The majority of those entering a nursing home stay less than one year, and one-third to one-half stay less than three months. Women are more likely than men of comparable age to enter a nursing home. Women of 85 years and older have a rate of nursing-home use per 1,000 population of 251, compared to 16 for women 65 to 74 and 81 for women 75 to 84. A similar pattern exists for men, although their utilization rates are lower.

In 1990 the Health Care Financing Administration published the second edition of a consumer guide to the nation's nursing homes entitled *Medicare/Medicaid Nursing Home Information.* State nursing-home ombudsmen, Medicaid offices, and all federally certified nursing homes have copies of the publication. The highly controversial guide evaluates nursing homes in every state by 32 criteria, ranging from the way food is stored to administration of drugs. Criticism of the report includes accusations that it does not distinguish between mild and serious problems and that it underrepresents civil-rights and abuse problems. However, consumers might want to check the guides to identify facilities that have a profusion of problems. A word of warning, however: not all facilities with problems will show up as red flags in the guide. The fact that a facility is not listed as having problems does not mean that it does not have them.

Who Pays for Nursing-Home Care

More than half of nursing-home costs for older residents are paid for by the individual or the family. *An important distinction between Medicaid and Medicare is that Medicaid will pay for care in a nursing home for those who meet low-income requirements, but Medicare does not pay for long-term care in nursing homes.* Medicare pays for less than 2 percent of nursing-home expenses, representing less than 1 percent of the total Medicare budget. And private insurance pays even less. After residents and their families, the dominant payer for nursing-home expenses is Medicaid. In 1987 Medicaid paid more than 42 percent of the nation's nursing-home expenses.

The Rights of Medicaid Patients in Nursing Homes

In 1987, the latest year for which data are available, Medicaid provided nursing-home benefits for 574,000 beneficiaries. There are several important points to take into consideration regarding Medicaid coverage for nursing-home costs:

Applicants to nursing homes *cannot* be required to pay money "up front" or to be a private-pay patient for a period of time before applying for Medicaid.

By law, nursing homes may *not* pressure family members into paying any money on behalf of a Medicaid resident.

Not all nursing-home services and items are covered by Medicaid. For example, Medicaid residents must pay for laundry services and nonprescription drugs themselves.

Transfer of Assets To Become Eligible for Medicaid

Some older people give away their assets to relatives so that they can meet Medicaid's eligibility requirements. Medicaid then pays the costs of care in a nursing home. Transfer of assets made after July 1, 1988, under these circumstances is subject to a new law that went into effect on that date. The law applies specifically to individuals who transfer assets for the purpose of entering a nursing home. Transfers made for people outside of institutions do not apply.

According to the law, if an individual transfers assets for less than fair market value within 30 months of application for public assistance, it would be assumed that they had transferred the assets for the purpose of becoming eligible for Medicaid, and the transfer could penalize the person in the nursing home. For example, if Mrs. Smith, an 81-year-old grandmother in need of nursing-home care, "sold" $150,000 worth of stock to her daughter and son-in-law for $5,000, moved into a nursing home, and 12 months later applied for Medicaid, it would be assumed that she was giving away her assets so that Medicaid would pick up the tab for her nursing-home bill.

The period of ineligibility depends on the value of the asset that was transferred. However, it cannot exceed 30 months. The law does not apply to the transfer of a home in the following circumstances:

When transferred to a spouse

When transferred to a dependent or disabled child

When transferred to a sibling with an equity interest in the home for one year prior to the Medicaid applicant's admission to a nursing home

When transferred to the child of the applicant who lived in the house for two years prior to admission to the nursing home and who had been a care giver to the nursing-home resident

There are also exceptions for the following types of asset transfer:

When the transfer is to an at-home spouse or blind or disabled child

When the applicant can prove that he or she intended to get fair market value

When the applicant can prove that the transfer was made for some purpose other than to qualify for Medicaid

When the denial of eligibility would result in undue hardship

States vary in the way they implement the law. Individuals who are planning to sell their home or reduce assets to apply for Medicaid would benefit from checking with a lawyer first.

Spousal Impoverishment Protection

The Medicare Catastrophic Coverage Act of 1988 included an important provision that supplied financial protection for spouses of nursing-home residents. Fortunately, the provision survived even though Congress repealed the act late in 1989. Since September 30, 1989, all states have been required to allow the spouse of a nursing-home resident who remains at home to keep *at least* a specified amount of income each month ($786 in 1989) and between $12,000 and $60,000 in liquid assets. Any liquid assets owned by either spouse are counted together and then proportioned equally. Any liquid assets in excess of the limit set by the state that belong to the spouse remaining at home are attributed to the institutionalized spouse, who must "spend down" until he or she meets Medicaid's eligibility requirements. The law allows states to increase the amount of income and assets that can be kept by the spouse at home.

Liens on the Property of Medicaid Patients in Nursing Homes

States have the option of putting a lien on the property of a nursing-home resident receiving assistance from Medicaid if his or her income is used for care. For states to put a lien on the resident's home, they must establish at a hearing that the person cannot reasonably be expected ever to return home. States may *not* put a lien on a resident's home in the following circumstances:

When the spouse is living in the home

When a child under age 21 is living in the home

When a blind or disabled child is living in the home

When a sibling with equity interest in the house has resided there for at least a year prior to the Medicaid recipient's entering a nursing home

States may also recover from the deceased's estate the cost of the Medicaid benefits that a deceased individual received.

Other Residential Options for Long-Term Care

Residences such as assisted-living centers and campus-like retirement communities are increasingly popular alternatives to nursing homes. Neither Medicaid nor Medicare will pay for such residences. However, other public programs provided through the Department of Housing and Urban Development assist low-income persons who qualify. For more information on such programs, see *Housing Options and Services for Older Adults: A Reference Handbook* in ABC-CLIO's Choices and Challenges series.

Long-Term-Care Insurance

Long-term-care insurance is designed to help cover the costs of nursing-home or home health care on a long-range basis. It is the new kid on the insurance-industry block, and there are major problems to be worked out before it is a viable alternative for older health consumers. A survey sponsored by the Robert Wood Johnson Foundation and conducted by Mark Mieners at the Maryland Center on Aging shows that many would like to purchase long-term-care insurance if good policies were available. The survey contacted 1,003 persons age 18 and over and found that 72 percent were willing to pay $50 a month for long-term-care insurance, and 55 percent were willing to pay $100 a month. Of those who did not want to pay for such insurance, almost a quarter said they disliked the available policies.

The majority favored having the government help buy long-term-care insurance. Unfortunately, several recent major reports by the Brookings Institution, United Seniors Health Cooperative, *Consumer Reports,* and the Families USA Foundation have been very critical of the majority of policies that are presently available to seniors. The problems:

Premiums are expensive in relation to benefits

Policies offer limited services

Benefits do not keep up with inflation

Policies usually exclude the very people who need the insurance most

According to Dr. Joshua Wiener, an expert on long-term care at the Brookings Institution: "The extent to which this type of insurance mechanism can reduce costs for both individuals and society is debatable." And James Firman, president of the United Seniors Health Cooperative, says: "It's like buying a home-owner's policy that would only pay to rebuild two rooms if the house burned down."

The cooperative did a study of 77 typical, private long-term insurance plans offered by 21 firms. While its analysis is controversial, some of the findings are worth considering:

Eighty percent of the plans have severe restrictions in coverage that make it difficult for policyholders to collect any benefits.

Seventy-seven percent won't pay nursing-home benefits unless the individual is first admitted to a hospital for the same condition; 54 percent of nursing-home patients don't qualify. The average probability of *not* collecting benefits is 61 percent if the individual is admitted to a nursing home.

Another study, by the Families USA Foundation, found that most older Americans cannot afford the cost of a basic nursing-home insurance policy. According to Families USA:

Seventy-three percent of all older Americans between the ages of 65 and 79 *cannot* afford to buy the lowest-priced nursing-home insurance policy that meets minimum standards

Eighty-four percent *cannot* afford to buy an average-priced policy

The older Americans are the more likely they *cannot* afford the average cost of nursing-home insurance

Some analysts insist that good long-term-care policies are presently available for those who can afford them, however. And most feel that better and better policies will come on the market. As of this writing, Congress is considering adopting long-term-care insurance protections similar to those now in effect for supplemental health insurance. It is worthwhile to watch the industry closely. Older health consumers who are interested in purchasing such policies should look over the checklist provided here and consult others that are available through such organizations as the United Seniors. However, a rule of thumb recommended by many analysts, including the staff of *Consumer Reports,* is that individuals with modest incomes should *not* purchase long-term-care insurance at all because they would quickly qualify for Medicaid benefits.

Types of Long-Term-Care Insurance Policies

The number of companies offering long-term-care policies increased from 16 in 1984 to 105 at the end of 1988. They include large companies such as Blue Cross and Blue Shield as well as smaller ones. As mentioned earlier, new types of coverage are coming on the market all the time. Some new products, for example, are not indemnity plans but cover a percentage of costs. Other new products offer unskilled care without requiring prior nursing-home care.

There are two types of long-term-care policies: "low" and "high" option. A typical low-option policy might, among other things, provide a $40-a-day reimbursement for skilled-nursing care at an annual cost of $318 for persons age 65 and $728 for those age 79 to 80. A high-option policy might provide $60 a day in reimbursement at a yearly cost of $684 for 65-year-olds and a staggering $1,496 for persons 79 to 80. Regardless of the type of policy an individual has, he or she should assume that at some point the premium will increase. Policy provisions for the length of coverage and deductibles also vary significantly. A low-option policy might provide coverage for only one year, while a high-option policy could provide coverage for up to six years. A low-option policy might have a deductible period of 90 to 100 days, and a high-option policy might have a deductible period of 20 days.

Another important area where these policies vary is in the types of services that they cover. While most policies offer nursing-home care, home care is included only about half the time, for example. All policies also reserve the right to exclude persons who are "high risk." High risk might be anything from cataracts to rare conditions such as Addison's disease. Insurers also usually will not sell policies to people over a certain age, and although half the policies now available can be purchased by people in their 80s, they are prohibitively expensive.

Regardless of the type of policy an older health consumer is interested in, he or she will be asked many personal questions when filling out an application. These questions are asked in order to determine the individual's risk of needing the services covered by the policy. High-risk persons will not get the coverage. It is important for beneficiaries to be very truthful when filling out the application, or the company may not pay benefits due to a condition not disclosed in the application.

What To Look For in Long-Term-Care Insurance

The long-term-care insurance industry is in a state of flux, with—it is hoped—improved policies on the horizon. For example, through funding from the Robert Wood Johnson Foundation, eight states are developing partnerships with private insurers to make long-term-care insurance affordable. The eight states are California, Connecticut, Indiana, Massachusetts, New Jersey, New York, Oregon, and Wisconsin. Under this program Massachusetts is considering a plan that would determine how much an individual could afford for long-term-care insurance, and the state would pick up the remaining cost.

Health consumers who are thinking about purchasing a long-term-care insurance policy should check the following:

- Is there a free-look provision, which means that an individual can return a policy within a certain period and have the premium and policy fee refunded?

- What is the actual coverage? Is the policy's reimbursement per day low? Forty dollars a day will not go far toward covering a $20,000-to-$25,000 yearly nursing-home bill.

- Is the policy guaranteed renewable? If not, it may be cancelable. This is not to your advantage, as this type of insurance is still essentially experimental. The California Department of Insurance recommends that no one consider buying a long-term-care insurance policy unless it is "guaranteed renewable for life."

- Has the policy a deductible or waiting period? This means that before the coverage will start, the individual has to pay his or her own way for a period of time.

- Look out for limitations and exclusions. Most policies have exclusions under which benefits will not be paid, for example, services outside the United States or in a federal facility.

- Check the policy's coverage restrictions. Does a doctor have to determine need? Does an individual have to have been hospitalized prior to using services? Are preexisting conditions such as Alzheimer's disease excluded? What is the deductible period?

- What is the policy's length of coverage?

- Where may care be provided? Skilled-nursing-facility coverage alone is too restrictive, for instance. Does the policy cover home health care? If not, it is not a good policy.

- Are there any period-of-confinement provisions? Such provisions stipulate how long the insured person can stay out of the nursing home before having to go through a new waiting period.

Life Insurance Options for Long-Term Care

A promising new concept in life insurance was just coming on the market as this was being written. Several life insurance companies, including Prudential Insurance Co. of America and Lincoln National Corporation, were offering policyholders the option of using the policy to pay for long-term medical care. The idea behind the policies is that rather than paying benefits when the insured dies, the policy will pay if the insured is in need of long-term care. Other similar policies will pay both death and long-term-care benefits. For example, under the Prudential plan insured persons who have been certified by a physician to have less than six months to live and nursing-home residents with no prospect of returning home would receive most of the value of the policy.

There are presently tax questions regarding these policies that must be settled in order for them to become widely available to consumers. And some states will not allow the sale of combined life and health policies. However, the concept is a promising one for health-care consumers.

Financing Long-Term Care through Home-Equity Conversion

Home-equity conversion is a creative new approach to long-term-care financing. Through home-equity conversion, a private lending institution gives money to the older homeowner and then recovers expenses when the home is sold. The resident can remain in the home while receiving cash payments, and the money can be used to purchase long-term care. There are many types of home-equity plans, and home-equity conversion is not for everyone. Under most circumstances, the plans are most helpful to people who are well above age 65 and who own their house free and clear.

For information on home-equity conversion, see *Housing Options and Services for Older Adults* in the ABC-CLIO Choices and Challenges series.

Chapter 8

Saving Health-Care Dollars

FACTS ON SAVING HEALTH-CARE DOLLARS

- Taxpayers should check to see whether they are eligible for medical-expense deductions and federal tax credits for dependent care to cut down on their federal tax liability.

- When a family member dies, no claim can be made against the family unless it has been agreed to in writing.

- Medicare encourages people to get second surgical opinions for costly medical procedures.

- Billions of dollars are spent every year on worthless, dangerous health treatments. For example, older health consumers should stay away from laetrile and chelation therapy clinics.

Introduction

This chapter is a potpourri of important consumer tips for cutting some of the fat out of health-care costs. The tips range from a list of health-promotion techniques recommended by the National Institute on Aging (NIA) to a description of medical-expense deductions for federal income tax.

Checklist for Reducing Health-Care Costs

The following is a summary of the pointers for reducing health-care costs described in this chapter. Other important consumer tips are interspersed throughout the first section of this book.

Practice health promotion

Obtain second opinions for costly medical procedures

Use less-expensive ambulatory facilities

Order generic drugs whenever possible

Make sure that all tests a doctor is having performed are medically necessary

Use medical deductions and tax credits for dependent care when they apply

If a relative other than a spouse has died, don't be talked into paying his or her bills for emotional reasons

Stay away from controversial therapies such as laetrile and chelation

Health-Promotion Techniques

The National Institute on Aging, a federal research agency that is part of the National Institutes of Health, suggests the following techniques for cutting down on health-care costs through staying healthy. Many of these tips are common sense, but because of their central role in keeping down costs through preventing disease, they cannot be emphasized enough.

Don't smoke

Eat a balanced diet and maintain your desired weight

Exercise regularly

Have regular health checkups, see a doctor when you detect a problem, and follow a doctor's advice when taking medications

Stay involved with family and friends

Allow time for rest and relaxation

Get enough sleep

Stay active through work, recreation, and community activities

Drink alcoholic beverages in moderation, if at all, and don't drive after drinking

Use seatbelts

Avoid overexposure to the sun and cold

Practice good safety habits at home to prevent accidents such as fires and falls

Medical-Expense Deductions for Federal Taxes

Medical-expense deductions on federal income taxes can benefit health consumers with modest incomes and large medical expenses. Any expenses that exceed 7.5 percent of adjusted gross income may be deducted. Individuals may deduct only that portion of their expenses that they alone were responsible for. They cannot deduct expenses that were reimbursed by Medicare or supplemental insurance. The following are deductible health expenses:

Prescription drugs and insulin (not over-the-counter drugs or vitamins).

Doctors' fees.

Hospital expenses (but not personal expenses).

Transportation to and from the doctor's or dentist's office or other place or treatment.

Medical-insurance premiums.

Medical supplies and equipment.

Certain lodging and meals away from home in connection with medical care.

Therapy and treatment of specific medical problems.

Care in a nursing home as long as medical care is one of the reasons for the stay. When residence in a nursing home is to provide assistance for a chronic problem, only the medical-care portion of the stay is deductible. Room and board are *not* deductible.

Drug-abuse and alcoholism clinics.

Home nursing care when connected with a physical disability or neurological disorder.

Deductions may be taken also for a range of expenses such as dentures, hearing aids, artificial limbs, Braille typewriters, and special telephones and other equipment for the deaf.

Federal Tax Credits for Dependent Care

Twenty-nine states now have some form of dependent-care tax credit. According to the Internal Revenue Service, 7.5 million households benefited from the credit in 1984. A small federal tax credit is also available for working people who provide care for dependents such as elderly parents. Individuals must meet all of the following requirements:

Husband and wife must be working or looking for work

The individual or couple filing the claim must be paying one-half of the household expenses

The expenses must be incurred to enable the person(s) filing the claim to work

And the older dependent person must be

A mentally or physically incapacitated person who is claimed as dependent

A spouse who is physically or mentally handicapped and unable to care for himself or herself

The following caps apply to the credit:

No more than $2,400 may be counted for one dependent and $4,800 for two or more dependents.

The deduction is limited to the amount of income earned by either spouse, whichever is lower. (Disabled spouses are treated as if they earned $200 per month.)

The deduction is limited to a percentage of income ranging from 20 to 30 percent.

When a Relative Dies

Often when a family member dies leaving large, unpaid medical bills, the family assumes they are responsible for these bills and takes on the debt for emotional reasons. However, according to the U.S. Senate Special Committee on Aging, unless an individual has agreed in writing to assume this financial responsibility, he or she is not liable. After a recipient of medical or hospital services has died, the hospital or doctor has a claim against his or her insurance and whatever part of the estate is allocated for these expenses by state law. No claim can be made against the family.

Second Surgical Opinions

Between 1971 and 1984 surgical procedures in the United States increased at a rate of growth that is four times the rate of population growth. Medicare encourages participants to get second surgical opinions whenever a doctor recommends surgery for a costly procedure (unless, of course, it is an emergency). Part B of Medicare will pay for a second opinion in the same way that it pays for other services. Medicare beneficiaries interested in getting a second opinion should call Medicare's Second Opinion Hotline, listed on page 173.

Ambulatory Emergency Centers

Most people would avoid checking into a hospital if there were a safe alternative. More than 2,000 walk-in centers in the United States provide quick, competent emergency care for relatively minor medical problems such as a broken bone or bad cold. Ambulatory centers may also be called emergi-centers or free-standing emergency centers. *Medicare beneficiaries should make sure that ambulatory centers are Medicare-certified before using their services.* Most walk-in centers can and do handle more severe emergencies, but that is not their specialty. At present there are no enforced standards for the industry. Some centers may be members of the Accreditation Association for Ambulatory Care or the Joint Commission on Accreditation of Hospitals, but accreditation is voluntary, and lack of it does not necessarily reflect inadequate care. Individuals who are going to have surgery performed in a walk-in center should schedule it for early in the morning so that they can spend the day recuperating at the center if they need to.

Saving Money on Prescription Drugs

Older Americans equal 12 percent of the nation's population but consume 25 percent of all prescriptions. In 1982 older adults were paying $93 a year for such medications. In addition, a recent report by the Congressional Budget Office states that 17 percent of Medicare Part B recipients spend more than $500 annually for their prescription drugs. Two other reports by the General Accounting Office reveal that *15.5 percent of older adults cannot pay for the prescriptions they require.*

The following provides tips on saving money on prescription drugs.

Locate drugstores that offer discounts to seniors. (Medicaid recipients should be sure to take their cards with them when they buy prescription drugs.)

Don't buy brand-name drugs. Order drugs by their generic or chemical names. According to the American Association of Retired Persons, generic drugs can save an average of 50 percent on the cost of a brand-name drug when purchased in quantities of 100. Some generics can save as much as 80 percent. However, if you do use a generic drug, make sure that your physician knows that it is generic.

When a physician approves, buy drugs in quantity.

Ask friends and medical professionals which pharmacies have the lowest prices. Ask physicians for sample medications to test before you buy a quantity.

Saving Money on Medical Care

The following tips will help older consumers save money on medical bills.

Make sure that all tests a physician is having performed are medically necessary. In some cases a second opinion may be needed.

Make sure that any surgery that is being scheduled is covered by Medicare and supplemental plans.

Question whether it is necessary to have all the medical treatment that is being scheduled in or out of the hospital.

Whenever possible, use providers who accept assignment.

Clinics and Doctors To Stay Away From

Both the congressional U.S. Senate Special Committee on Aging and the House Select Committee on Aging have conducted extensive studies on medical fraud and have found that billions of dollars are spent every year on worthless, dangerous health treatments. The following is a list of hospitals and clinics it is advisable to avoid:

Cancer clinics that promote unproved therapies

Laetrile clinics

Chelation therapy clinics

Arthritis clinics

The directors and staffs of these clinics often use misleading initials after their names to convince the unwary that they are at least semilegitimate. Examples are N.D. (Doctor of Neuropathy) and Ms.D. (Doctor of Metaphysics). These initials do not describe medical doctors who are qualified to treat medical problems.

Sources for Part One

American Association of Retired Persons. *Changing Needs for Long-Term Care: A Chartbook*. Washington, DC: 1989.

Families USA Foundation and United Seniors Health Cooperative. *The Unaffordability of Nursing Home Insurance*. Washington, DC: Families USA Foundation, 1990.

Friedman, Jo-Ann. *Home-Health Care*. New York: Norton, 1986.

Gelfand, Donald E. *The Aging Network*. New York: Springer, 1988.

Health Care Financing Administration. *The Medicare Handbook*. Washington, DC: U.S. Government Printing Office, March 15, 1989.

Hellman, Susan. *Medicare, Medigap and Other Impossible Things Revealed*. Denver: Colorado Gerontological Society, 1989.

Huttman, Elizabeth. *Social Services for the Elderly*. New York: The Free Press, 1985.

Roberts, Ralph. *The Veterans Guide to Benefits*. New York: New American Library, 1989.

Spitzner-Reznick, Jeffrey. *Your Real Medicare Handbook*. Madison, WI: Center for Public Representation, 1987.

U.S. Congress. Committee on Ways and Means. *Background Material and Data on Programs within the Jurisdiction of the Committee on Ways and Means*. Washington, DC: U.S. Government Printing Office.

U.S. Senate. Special Committee on Aging, in conjunction with the American Association of Retired Persons, the Federal Council on Aging, and the Administration on Aging. *Aging America, Trends and Projections*, 1987–1988 and 1989–1990 eds. Washington, DC: U.S. Government Printing Office.

U.S. Senate. Special Committee on Aging. *Developments in Aging: 1987, Volume One*. Washington, DC: U.S. Government Printing Office, 1988.

Waldo, Daniel R., Sally T. Sonnefeld, David R. McKusick, and Ross H. Arnett III. "Health Expenditures by Age Group, 1977 and 1987," *Health Care Financing Review*, Summer 1989, 111–120.

Williams, Stephen J., and Paul R. Torrens. *Introduction to Health Services*, 3rd ed. New York: John Wiley and Sons, 1988.

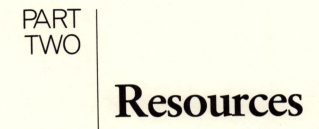

PART
TWO

Resources

The second part of *Paying for Health Care after Age 65* is a handy, selective directory of organizations and reference materials. It includes a comprehensive list of state publications and organizations as well as national resources.

This book was finished late in 1989, when the Medicare Catastrophic Coverage Act had just been repealed. Owing to the repeal, many of the sources that were planned for inclusion in Chapter 11 became outdated and had to be deleted. A number of these publications will certainly be updated, and other new books explaining Medicare's coverage will be published in the near future.

Chapter 9

Who's Who in Health Care

Older persons may be treated by a number of professionals in a number of settings. With the great variety of health providers, it is important for beneficiaries to understand which professionals can offer the best and least costly care for a specific problem and which services normally will be paid for by Medicare. The following brief index covers the majority of the medical practitioners frequently seen by older people, and it identifies whether their services are covered by Medicare.

General Medical Care

Doctors of Medicine (M.D.s) treat diseases and injuries, provide preventive care, do routine checkups, prescribe drugs, and perform some surgery. M.D.s complete medical school plus three to seven years of graduate medical education. They must be licensed in the state in which they practice. *Their services are covered by Medicare.*

Internists (M.D.s) are M.D.s who specialize in the diagnosis and medical treatment of disease in adults. Internists do not perform surgery or deliver babies. *Their services are covered by Medicare.*

Family Practitioners (M.D.s) are M.D.s who specialize in providing comprehensive health care for all members of a family, regardless of age or sex, on a continuing basis. *Their services are covered by Medicare.*

153

Doctors of Osteopathic Medicine (D.O.s) provide general health care to individuals and families. The training they receive is similar to that of an M.D. In addition to drugs, surgery, and other treatments, a D.O. may manipulate muscles and bones to treat specific problems.

Medical Specialists (M.D.s) treat specific areas:

Cardiologists—heart

Dermatologists—skin

Endocrinologists—glands of internal secretion, such as diabetes

Gastroenterologists—digestive tract

Gynecologists—female reproductive system

Neurologists—nervous system

Oncologists—tumors and cancer

Ophthalmologists—eyes

Orthopedists—bones, muscles, ligaments, and tendons

Rheumatologists—arthritis and rheumatism

Urologists—urinary system

Most of the services of these specialists are covered by Medicare.

Physician Assistants (P.A.s) are most often seen in doctors' offices or hospitals doing some of the tasks traditionally performed by doctors. They give physical examinations, take medical histories, carry out diagnostic tests, and develop treatment plans for patients. Their education includes two to four years of college, followed by a two-year period of special training. P.A.s must always be under the supervision of a doctor, but, depending on state laws, the supervision can be by telephone rather than in person. In some states P.A.s can prescribe certain drugs. *Medicare will pay for the services provided by the P.A. only if they are performed in a hospital or doctor's office under the supervision of a doctor.*

Nurse Practitioners (R.N.s, N.P.s) are registered nurses with training beyond basic nursing education. Nurse practitioners perform physical examinations and diagnostic tests, counsel patients, and develop treatment programs. Regulations regarding their duties vary from state to state. Nurse practitioners may work independently, such as in rural clinics, or may be staff members at hospitals and other health facilities. *Medicare will help pay for nurse-practitioner services performed under the supervision of a doctor.*

Registered Nurses (R.N.s) may have two, three, or four years of education in a nursing school. In addition to performing bedside nursing duties, such as giving medicine, administering treatments, and educating patients, R.N.s also work in doctors' offices, clinics, and community health agencies. *Medicare does not cover private-duty nursing. It helps to pay for general nursing services by reimbursing hospitals, skilled-nursing facilities, and home health agencies for part of the nurses' salaries.*

Dental Care

Dentists (D.D.S.s or D.M.D.s) treat oral conditions such as gum disease and tooth decay. They do regular checkups, give routine dental and preventive care, fill cavities, remove teeth, provide dentures, and check for cancers of the mouth. Dentists can prescribe medication and perform oral surgery. A general dentist might refer patients to a specialist such as an oral surgeon, who does difficult tooth removals and surgery on the jaw; an endodontist, who is an expert on root canals; or a periodontist, who is especially knowledgeable about gum diseases. *Medicare will not pay for any dental care except for surgery on the jaw or facial bones.*

Dental Hygienists (R.D.H.s) examine, clean, and polish teeth. They also take X rays and teach patients about proper dental care. Although hygienists' duties vary according to state law, they almost always work under the supervision of a dentist. Most hygienists have a least two years of formal training, and all are licensed by the state in which they practice. *Medicare does not pay for their services.*

Dental Assistants help dentists and dental hygienists in the dental office. They may process X rays, prepare the patient for examination, schedule appointments, or assist the dentist while he or she works. Dental assistants may have some formal training, or they may learn their responsibilities on the job. *Their services are not covered by Medicare.*

Eye Care

Ophthalmologists (M.D.s) are M.D.s who specialize in the diagnosis and treatment of diseases of the eye. They also prescribe eyeglasses and contact lenses. Like other M.D.s., ophthalmologists can prescribe drugs and perform surgery. They often treat older people who have glaucoma and cataracts. *Medicare helps pay for all medically necessary surgery or treatment of eye diseases and for examinations and eyeglasses to correct vision after cataract surgery. But it will not pay for routine examinations, eyeglasses, or contact lenses.*

Optometrists (O.D.s) have a bachelor's degree plus three years of training in a school of optometry. They are trained to prescribe, supply, and adjust eyeglasses and contact lenses. Although optometrists cannot prescribe drugs, in some states they are allowed to use certain drugs in their offices. An optometrist refers patients to an ophthalmologist for more-complicated diagnosis or treatment, or for care requiring medication or surgery. *Medicare pays for only a limited number of optometric visits.*

Opticians fit, supply, and adjust eyeglasses and contact lenses prescribed by an ophthalmologist or optometrist. They cannot examine or test the eye, or prescribe glasses or drugs. Opticians are licensed in about half the states and may have formal training. Traditionally, however, most opticians learn their skills during on-the-job training. *Their services are not covered by Medicare* with the exception of supplying eyeglasses to correct vision after cataract surgery.

Muscle, Bone, and Foot Care

Orthopedists (M.D.s or D.O.s) are surgeons who operate on and treat problems of the bones, joints, muscles, ligaments, and tendons. *Medicare does pay for their services.*

Chiropractors are not medical doctors but manipulate the spine to restore normal functioning to diseased systems. *Medicare pays only for the manual manipulation of the spine to correct a specific problem that can be demonstrated by X ray. Medicare will not pay for the diagnostic or therapeutic services of a chiropractor.*

Podiatrists (D.P.M.s) diagnose, treat, and prevent diseases and injuries of the foot. They may do surgery, make devices to correct or prevent foot problems, provide toenail care, and prescribe certain drugs. A podiatrist is not licensed to treat diseases or injuries of any other part of the body. Podiatrists complete four years of professional school, and once they have been licensed *Medicare will cover the cost of their services except for routine foot care. (However, routine foot care is covered if it is necessary because of diabetic complications.)*

Mental-Health Care

Psychiatrists (M.D.s) are M.D.s who treat people with mental and emotional difficulties. They can prescribe medication and counsel patients, as well as perform diagnostic tests to determine if there are physical problems. *Medicare will pay for a portion of both inpatient and outpatient psychiatric costs.*

Psychologists (Ph.D.s) are not medical doctors but are called doctor because they have a doctoral degree in psychology. They counsel people with mental and emotional problems. *The services of a clinical psychologist are not covered by Medicare except when they are performed in connection with the services of an M.D. or a psychiatrist.*

Other Medical Care

Registered Dietitians (R.D.s) provide nutritional care and dietary counseling. Most of them work in hospitals or doctors' offices, but some have private practices. R.D.s complete a bachelor's degree and an internship (or an approved coordinated undergraduate program), they also pass an examination. *Medicare generally will not pay for a dietitian's services. However, it does reimburse hospitals and skilled-nursing facilities for a portion of dietitians' salaries.*

Physical Therapists (P.T.s) help people whose strength, ability to move, sensation, or range of motion is impaired. They may use exercise; heat, cold, or water therapy; or other treatments to control pain, strengthen muscles, and improve coordination. All P.T.s complete a program leading to a bachelor's degree, and some receive postgraduate training. Patients are usually referred by a doctor, and *Medicare pays some of the costs of outpatient treatments. Physical therapy performed in a hospital or skilled-nursing facility is covered by Medicare.*

Occupational Therapists (O.T.s) assist patients with handicaps to function more independently. They may provide exercise programs; heat, cold, or whirlpool treatments to relieve pain; and hand splints and adaptive equipment to improve function and independence. O.T.s have a bachelor's degree plus six months' specialized training. *The costs of occupational therapy will be paid in part by Medicare if the patient is referred as an outpatient by a doctor, or in full if the patient is in a hospital or skilled-nursing facility.*

Speech-Language Pathologists are concerned with speech and language problems, and *audiologists* are involved with hearing disorders. Some specialists work in both areas. They test and evaluate patients, and they plan therapy to restore as much normal function as possible. Many speech-language pathologists work with stroke victims, those who have dementia, patients with diseases of the nervous system, and people who have had their vocal cords removed. Many audiologists work with older people whose hearing may be failing. They recommend hearing aids when they are needed and sometimes dispense them. Speech-language pathologists have at least a master's degree. Most of them are licensed by the state in which they practice. *Medicare generally will cover the services of speech-language pathologists and audiologists.*

Social Workers in health-care settings alert patients to community services that might be useful, arrange for counseling when necessary, and help patients and their families handle problems related to physical and mental illness and disability. Older people might be referred to social workers by various health providers or their local governments. A social worker's education may include a master's degree (M.S.W.). *Medicare does not cover services provided by social workers unless they work in a hospital setting.*

Homemaker—Home Health Aides provide personal care such as assistance in bathing, grooming, dressing, cooking, and cleaning under the supervision of a professional. Standards for these services are set by the National Council for Homemaker—Home Health Aide Services. *Medicare will cover these services only when the beneficiary's health status meets the home health care benefit guidelines.*

Chapter 10

Directory of Organizations

General Organizations

American Association of Retired Persons (AARP)
Horace B. Deets, Executive Director
1909 K Street, NW
Washington, DC 20049
(202) 872-4700

By far the largest of the aging organizations, AARP is a non-profit, nonpartisan organization with 27 million members age 50 and above. AARP's goals are to promote independence, dignity, and purpose for older persons in society, and to improve the image of aging. AARP has 3,400 local chapters. The organization offers a wide range of books and pamphlets that address issues of interest to older people. Members receive a bimonthly magazine, *Modern Maturity,* and a newsletter. AARP also offers members a number of types of insurance. However, as with any insurance policy, AARP'S coverage should be carefully compared to other policies before it is purchased.

AARP's Health Advocacy Services (HAS) is an AARP program that among other things encourages effective use of the health-care system. HAS runs the Medicare/Medicaid Assistance Project (MMAP), which provides guidance to older persons so that they can use Medicare and Medicaid effectively. MMAP is active in a number of states where volunteers provide assistance on Medicare claims and appeals.

American Bar Association Commission on Legal Problems of the Elderly

Nancy Coleman, Staff Director
1800 M Street, NW
Washington, DC 20036
(202) 331-2200

> The American Bar Association established the 15-member inter-
> disciplinary Commission on Legal Problems of the Elderly in
> 1978 to analyze and respond to the law-related needs of older
> people in the United States. The commission has focused on a
> number of issues important to health-care costs such as long-term
> care and health-care decision-making. The commission provides
> information and guidance in areas of the law and seeks to gener-
> ate pro bono, reduced-fee, and community education programs
> for older persons, as well as relevant continuing legal-education
> programs for attorneys. The commission also publishes several
> documents on the law and aging, many of which are free.

Brookdale Center on Aging

Rose Dobraf, Executive Director
Institute on Law and Rights of Older Adults
Hunter College
425 East 25th Street
New York, NY 10010
(212) 481-4422

> The Institute on Law and Rights of Older Adults is a resource
> center for professionals working on entitlement programs such
> as Medicare and Medicaid. The center provides telephone con-
> sultation for anyone working on these issues and offers training
> in New York State. It publishes a free quarterly newsletter, the
> *Senior Rights Reporter,* which focuses on issues of entitlements
> for the elderly, and it issues bulletins on special topics. The center
> also has mimeographed materials and articles that are available
> to the public, as well as medigap and long-term care checklists.
> A publications list is available.

The Center for Public Representation (CPR)

Betsy Abramson, Director of Elderly Projects
520 University Avenue
Madison, WI 53703
(608) 251-4008

CPR is a nonprofit corporation that is a combination law firm, training center, watchdog, and publishing house, whose mission is to speak up for the unrepresented. CPR performs a long list of impressive activities, including representing elderly persons who lack access to quality health care. The center has a fourfold program of advocacy, research, consumer education, and training. While many activities are based in Wisconsin, several of the center's activities reach outside the state. For example, CPR contracts with the American Association of Retired Persons to train volunteer health-insurance counselors on Medicare, supplemental health insurance, and Medicaid. The center and AARP will be publishing a newspaper for volunteers. CPR offers a number of publications of interest to older health consumers, such as *Your Real Medicare Handbook*. A publications list is available.

ElderMed America (EMA)
Roberta Suber, Executive Vice-President
20500 Nordhoff Street
Chatsworth, CA 91311
(818) 407-2221

EMA is the parent company of two wholly owned subsidiaries that develop products for older persons, ElderMed Ventures and the ElderMed Institute. A membership organization for persons age 50 and older, EMA has members in 25 states. Two primary concerns are access to health care and health-care costs. EMA has a number of nationwide programs, including Medicare and insurance-claims assistance and counseling and mail-order pharmacy services. ElderMed offers members Medicare supplemental insurance, which, like any insurance policy, should be compared to other policies before it is purchased.

Families USA Foundation
(formerly Villers Foundation)
Phyllis Torda, Health Policy Director
1334 G Street, NW
Washington, DC 20005
(202) 628-3030

Formerly the Villers Foundation, the Families USA Foundation focuses its efforts on the needs of the low-income elderly, particularly in the areas of health care and income security. One of its interests is working to extend Medicaid to all of the elderly poor. The foundation provides funding for health-care campaigns and projects that benefit the low-income elderly, such as the Action Alliance Research and Education Program in Philadelphia, which, among other things, encourages doctors to accept Medicare assignment.

Health Insurance Association of America (HIAA)
Melanie Marsh, Manager of Public Affairs
1750 K Street, NW
Washington, DC 20006
(202) 223-7780; (800) 635-1271

Representing approximately 350 insurance companies, HIAA is a trade organization involved in lobbying for concerns of its members. It provides public information and produces several booklets on long-term care and medigap insurance. Publications are free and available by writing to P.O. Box 41455, Washington, DC 20018.

Intergovernmental Health Policy Project (IHPP)
Richard Merrit, Director
2011 I Street, NW, Suite 200
Washington, DC 20006
(202) 872-1445

IHPP is a university-based program concentrating its research efforts exclusively on the health laws and programs of the 50 states. It provides assistance to state executive officials, legislators, legislative staff, and others who need to know about important developments in other states. IHPP also helps federal officials identify innovative state health programs and specific state programs. Among other things, IHPP publishes *State Health Notes,* a monthly newsletter that focuses entirely on the health-related activities of state governments. *State Health Notes* is a particularly valuable source of information on state Medicaid programs. For subscription information, write John Sulsa at the above address. A publications list is available.

Legal Counsel for the Elderly (LCE)
Wayne Moore, Director

1331 H Street, NW, Room 1005
Washington, DC 20005
(202) 234-0970

The Legal Counsel for the Elderly is a free legal service to help Washington-area residents age 60 and older with such legal issues as problems with Medicaid and Medicare benefits. The organization helps clients directly or finds them attorneys. It also serves as a national legal support center. LCE's particularly well informed staff will answer telephone inquiries for those out of the area. The staff also produces a number of excellent publications on health-related issues, among them a protective-services manual, a disability manual, and a public-benefits checklist for Washington residents. LCE is establishing a legal-hotline service that will expand to all 50 states. Contact LCE for an updated publications list.

Other important projects of the LCE:

The National Training Project: LCE has trained more than 1,500 legal-services and aging advocates, including lawyers, paralegals, lay advocates, and volunteers. Topics in the training include Medicare, Nursing Home Law, and Protective Services.

National Support in Protective Services Law: LCE provides assistance to legal-services workers in the area of protective-services law.

Representative Payee Project: This project recruits volunteers to help manage the financial affairs of incapable older persons. Projects are currently operating in 31 sites in ten states and the District of Columbia.

National Library Project: Through LCE the American Association of Retired Persons National Gerontology Resource Center has expanded its collection of legal materials that are now available for free loan by mail. Lists of the materials and instructions for obtaining a loan are available from John Hortum at the above address and phone number.

Legal Services Corporation (LSC)
John H. Bayly, President and Chief Executive Officer

400 Virginia Avenue, SW
Washington, DC 20024-2751
(202) 863-1839

> LSC is a private, nonprofit organization, established by the Legal Services Corporation Act of 1974. The corporation funds more than 1,000 offices providing legal assistance to individuals with low incomes. One of its priorities is to provide legal services to the low-income elderly. LSC lawyers and paralegals often help elderly clients with Medicare appeals and problems with Medicaid benefits. To qualify for services, individuals must meet low-income requirements. LSC offices provide legal help in civil matters only and not in criminal matters.

The Long Term Care Campaign
Stephen McConnell, Coordinator
1334 G Street, NW, Third Floor
Washington, DC 20005
(202) 737-6340

> The Long Term Care Campaign is a coalition of more than 125 national organizations dedicated to enacting comprehensive legislation to protect U.S. families against the costs of long-term care. Along with drawing national attention to the issue, the campaign focuses its efforts in state legislatures. It highlights such issues as family care givers and the need for a national plan to help individuals pay their long-term-care bills. Local and state coalitions work with the organization to locate witnesses for hearings and to draw attention to its work. The campaign makes available printed materials and a video for use by groups for public education. Fact sheets published by the campaign include "What Experts Are Saying about Private Long-Term Care Insurance," "Facts About Caregivers," and "What Is Long-Term Care?"

National Association of Insurance Commissioners (NAIC)
Tim Brown, Public Relations
120 West Twelfth Street, Suite 1100
Kansas City, MO 64105
(816) 842-3600

> NAIC is a national trade organization representing each of the state insurance regulatory offices. Its members are state insurance commissioners or their representatives. The association has

two task forces important to older adults. The task force on supplemental health insurance codeveloped a buyer's guide on Medicare supplemental insurance (with the Health Care Financing Administration) and minimum guidelines for Medicare supplements. The long-term-care insurance task force has developed minimum guidelines for long-term-care insurance. NAIC also has a solvency-monitoring service for states in which it takes a broad-brush look at the financial status of insurance companies. Unfortunately, NAIC does not make this information available to the public. NAIC is a valuable resource for information on federal legislation and policy development in the area of health insurance for the elderly, as well as what is happening in individual states.

For a list of all the state divisions of insurance that are also members of the NAIC, see the following section on government agencies.

National Citizens Coalition for Nursing Home Reform (NCCNHR)
Elma Holder, Executive Director
1424 Sixteenth Street, NW, Suite L2
Washington, DC 20036
(202) 797-0657

NCCNHR has 250-plus member groups, which engage in a variety of activities relating to nursing homes and nursing-home costs, including promoting community involvement in nursing homes; assisting in resolving individual complaints and problems; collaborating with health-care workers to improve care in nursing homes; monitoring regulatory activities; and supporting resident and family councils. Recently NCCNHR successfully coordinated a national effort to achieve, in December 1987, the most comprehensive federal nursing-home reforms in more than a decade. The NCCNHR Clearinghouse publishes a bimonthly newsletter, the *Quality Care Advocate*. It also has a publications list of various topics it offers.

National Consumer League
Linda Golodner, Executive Director
815 Fifteenth Street, NW, Suite 516
Washington, DC 20005
(202) 639-8140

The National Consumer League is currently working with a coalition of other organizations to produce a newsletter for consumers who are selecting long-term-care services. It also publishes a free brochure called "Financing Long-Term Care—A Search for the Solution" and a fact sheet on Medicare. The league is updating their *Medicare Handbook* for older health consumers.

National Council of Senior Citizens (NCSC)
Lawrence T. Smedley, Executive Director
925 Fifteenth Street, NW
Washington, DC 20005
(202) 347-8800

NCSC is a leading nonprofit advocacy organization that works for human dignity for people of all ages. The National Council's 4.5-million membership includes 4,800 clubs across the country. NCSC has actively worked for issues such as long-term care, nursing-home reform, and national health care. NCSC has a monthly publication, *Senior Citizens News,* which informs members of current legislative happenings. It also publishes an annual *Congressional Voting Record* of concern to older adults, including such issues as Medicare, Medicaid, and supplemental health insurance.

National Council on the Aging, Inc. (NCOA)
Dr. David Thursz, Executive Director
600 Maryland Avenue, SW, West Wing 100
Washington, DC 20024
(202) 479-1200

The National Council on the Aging is a membership organization, primarily of professionals, that is active in seven major issues affecting the quality of life for older Americans: employment, rural aging, senior centers, senior housing, adult day care, community-based long-term care, and voluntary organizations. It is a national resource center for information, training, technical assistance, advocacy efforts, publications, and research relating to all aspects of aging, including health care and health-care costs. NCOA has seven professional membership units that correspond with its issue areas, including the National Institute of Senior Centers, the National Institute on Community-Based

Long Term Care, and the National Institute on Adult Day Care. NCOA publishes a number of books on health and related issues such as *Health Promotion and Aging: A National Directory of Selected Programs*.

National Health Law Program (NHLP)
Larry Levin, Director
2639 South La Cienega Boulevard
Los Angeles, CA 90034
Main Office (213) 204-6010; in Washington, DC (202) 887-5310

> NHLP represents low-income persons in seeking access to or financing for health care. Clients are representative of all age groups. Services include answering written and telephoned requests regarding Medicare, Medicaid, and related programs; immigrant rights to health care; publications development; community education; policy analysis; and research. The organization's staff will provide training in Medicare, Medicaid, and related programs at no charge to recipients in any area of the country.

National Senior Citizens Law Center (NSCLC)
Neil Dudovitz, Deputy Director
1052 West Sixth Street
Los Angeles, CA 90016
(213) 482-3550

> The National Senior Citizens Law Center was established in 1972 to help older Americans live their lives in dignity and freedom from poverty. NSCLC attorneys are conversant with a broad range of legal areas that affect the security and welfare of older persons of limited income. NSCLC staff primarily lend assistance to attorneys and paralegals in field programs funded by the Legal Services Corporation or the Administration on Aging. NSCLC offers technical assistance with Medicare claims and appeals and with litigation assistance on procedural issues. Assistance is also available on Medigap issues and Medicare-Medicaid dual-eligibility issues. The center also litigates against state and federal authorities to expand Medicaid eligibility and scope of benefits.

Older Women's League (OWL)
Laura Loeb, Director of Public Policy

1325 G Street, NW
Washington, DC 20005
(202) 783-6686

> The Older Women's League is the first national membership organization to focus solely on the concerns of midlife and older women. OWL is a nonprofit organization with 15,000 members and more than 100 chapters throughout the United Sates. A major focus is on continuation of health insurance after divorce, a spouse's death, or unemployment. OWL's easy-to-read publication, *Health Insurance Continuation,* provides important information about health insurance for workers and the unemployed. A publications list is available.

United Seniors Health Cooperative (USHC)
Chuck Mondin, Marketing Manager
1334 G Street, NW, Suite 500
Washington, DC 20005
(202) 393-6222

> USHC is a nonprofit membership organization providing health-care cost and benefit information to older consumers. It is the only aging-related organization that is focusing its efforts entirely in the area of health-care costs and related benefits. The organization arranges group buying plans, provides consumer information on issues such as long-term-care insurance, and helps people get the most from public benefits. USHC offers software programs, a newsletter, and publications to organizations and individuals.

Washington Business Group on Health (WBGH)
Willis Goldbeck, President
229¹/₂ Pennsylvania Avenue
Washington, DC 20003
(202) 547-6644

> The goal of the Washington Business Group on Health is to bring business and government closer together on health-policy concerns. Its Institute on Aging, Work, and Health serves as an information clearinghouse for employers on such issues as retiree health, health-care delivery, and long-term care. WBGH's publications include *Health Benefits for an Aging Workforce* and *Together on Aging.*

Government Agencies

Department of Veterans Affairs (VA)
Edward J. Derivinski, Secretary
810 Vermont Avenue, NW
Washington, DC 20024
(202) 233-4000

> The Department of Veterans Affairs, formerly the Veterans Administration, offers a number of programs providing assistance to veterans. Disability compensation and free or low-cost medical care are of particular importance to older veterans who are eligible for benefits. The department operates more than 150 hospitals across the country and many outpatient clinics.

Federal Information Centers (FICs)

> Older consumers who would like assistance in locating federal offices with information about services, programs, or regulations should contact the closest FIC listed below.

Alabama
Birmingham (205) 322-8591
Mobile (205) 438-1421

Alaska
Anchorage (907) 271-3650

Arizona
Phoenix (602) 261-3313

Arkansas
Little Rock (501) 378-6177

California
Los Angeles (213) 894-3800
Sacramento (916) 551-2380
San Diego (619) 557-6030
San Francisco (415) 556-6600
Santa Ana (714) 836-2386

Colorado
Colorado Springs
   (719) 471-9491
Denver (303) 844-6575
Pueblo (719) 544-9523

Connecticut
Hartford (203) 527-2617
New Haven (203) 624-4720

Florida
Ft. Lauderdale (305) 522-8531
Jacksonville (904) 354-4756
Miami (305) 536-4155
Orlando (305) 422-1800
St. Petersburg (813) 893-3495
Tampa (813) 229-7911
West Palm Beach
   (305) 833-7566

Georgia
Atlanta (404) 331-6891

Hawaii
Honolulu (808) 551-1365

Illinois
Chicago (312) 353-4242

Indiana
Gary (219) 883-4110
Indianapolis (317) 269-7373

Iowa
From all points in Iowa
(800) 532-1556 (toll-free)

Kansas
From all points in Kansas
(800) 432-2934 (toll-free)

Kentucky
Louisville (502) 582-6261

Louisiana
New Orleans (504) 589-6696

Maryland
Baltimore (301) 962-4980

Massachusetts
Boston (617) 565-8121

Michigan
Detroit (313) 226-7016
Grand Rapids (616) 451-2628

Minnesota
Minneapolis (612) 370-3333

Missouri
St. Louis (314) 425-4106
From elsewhere in Missouri
(800) 392-7711 (toll-free)

Nebraska
Omaha (402) 221-3353
From elsewhere in Nebraska
(800) 642-8383 (toll-free)

New Jersey
Newark (201) 645-3600
Trenton (609) 396-4400

New Mexico
Albuquerque (505) 766-3091

New York
Albany (518) 463-4421
Buffalo (716) 846-4010
New York (212) 264-4464
Rochester (716) 546-5075
Syracuse (315) 476-8545

North Carolina
Charlotte (704) 376-3600

Ohio
Akron (216) 375-5638
Cincinnati (513) 684-2801
Cleveland (216) 522-4040
Columbus (614) 221-1014
Dayton (513) 223-7377
Toledo (419) 241-3223

Oklahoma
Oklahoma City (405) 231-4868
Tulsa (918) 584-4193

Oregon
Portland (503) 221-2222

Pennsylvania
Philadelphia (215) 597-7042
Pittsburgh (412) 644-3456

Rhode Island
Providence (401) 331-5565

Tennessee
Chattanooga (615) 265-8231
Memphis (901) 521-3285
Nashville (615) 242-5056

Texas
Austin (512) 472-5494
Dallas (214) 767-8585
Fort Worth (817) 334-3624
Houston (713) 229-2552
San Antonio (512) 224-4471

Utah
Salt Lake City (801) 524-5353

Virginia
Norfolk (804) 441-3101
Richmond (804) 643-4928
Roanoke (703) 982-8591

Washington
Seattle (206) 442-0570
Tacoma (206) 383-5230

Wisconsin
Milwaukee (414) 271-2273

Health Care Financing Administration (HCFA)
Department of Health and Human Services
Denny Siebert, Director of Public Affairs
200 Independence Avenue, SW
Hubert Humphrey Building, Room 314 G
Washington, DC 20201
(202) 245-6726
Medicare Hotline: (800) 888-1770
Medicare Second Opinion Referral Center: (800) 638-6833; in Maryland
(800) 492-6603

> HCFA manages the Medicare and Medicaid programs and related medical-care quality control. The national office oversees district offices throughout the United States. It also contracts with many organizations across the country to handle claims for Medicare benefits. HCFA is responsible for providing beneficiaries with information about the programs it oversees through such aids as *The Medicare Handbook,* which is produced every year. HCFA publishes numerous pamphlets with information on every aspect of national health programs and operates a Medicare Hotline, which provides specifics about the Medicare program. HCFA's publications are distributed through local Social Security offices.

Insurance Commissions

> Each state has a division that regulates all insurance companies in that state, and these divisions are usually members of the National Association of Insurance Commissioners (NAIC). Commissions are responsible for licensing insurance companies and agents and for collecting premium taxes and fees. They also act as liaisons between consumers and the insurance industry and handle arbitration of consumer complaints regarding insurance companies. The addresses and phone numbers of NAIC-member state insurance divisions are listed below.

Alabama
135 South Union Street, No. 160
Montgomery, AL 36130-3401
(205) 269-3550

Alaska
P.O. Box "D"
Juneau, AK 99811
(907) 465-2515
FAX (907) 463-3841

American Samoa
Office of the Governor
Pago Pago, American Samoa 96797
(684) 633-4116

Arizona
3030 North Third Street, Suite 1100
Phoenix, AZ 85012
(602) 255-5400

Arkansas
400 University Tower Building
Twelfth and University Streets
Little Rock, AR 72204
(501) 371-1325
FAX (501) 371-5723

California
100 Van Ness Avenue
San Francisco, CA 94102
(415) 557-9624
FAX (415) 557-3076

Colorado
303 West Colfax Avenue,
  5th Floor
Denver, CO 80204
(303) 620-4300

Connecticut
165 Capitol Avenue
State Office Building, Room 425
Hartford, CT 06106
(203) 566-5275
FAX (203) 566-7410

Delaware
841 Silverlake Boulevard
Dover, DE 19901
(302) 736-4251
FAX (302) 736-5280

District of Columbia
613 G Street, NW,
  6th Floor
Washington, DC 20001
(202) 727-5422

Florida
Attention: Kim Forester
State Capitol
Plaza Level Eleven
Tallahassee, FL 32399-0300
(904) 488-3440
FAX (904) 488-0699

Georgia
2 Martin L. King, Jr., Drive
Floyd Memorial Building
704 West Tower
Atlanta, GA 30334
(404) 656-2056

Guam
855 West Marine Drive
P.O. Box 2796
Agana, Guam 96910
(011-671) 477-1040
FAX (011-671) 472-2643

Hawaii
P.O. Box 3614
Honolulu, HI 96811
(808) 548-5450
FAX (808) 548-2028

Idaho
500 South 10th Street
Boise, ID 83720
(208) 334-2250

Illinois
320 West Washington Street, 4th Floor
Springfield, IL 62767
(217) 782-4515
FAX (217) 782-5020
Chicago FAX (312) 917-5435

Indiana
311 West Washington Street, Suite 300
Indianapolis, IN 46204-2787
(317) 232-2386
FAX (317) 232-3548

Iowa
Lucas State Office Building, 6th Floor
Des Moines, IA 50319
(515) 281-5705
FAX (515) 281-3059

Kansas
420 SW Ninth Street
Topeka, KS 66612
(913) 296-7801
FAX (913) 296-2283

Kentucky
229 West Main Street
P.O. Box 517
Frankfort, KY 40602
(502) 564-3630
FAX (502) 223-4011

Louisiana
950 North Fifth Street
P.O. Box 94214
Baton Rouge, LA 70804-9214
(504) 342-5328
FAX (504) 342-3078

Maine
State Office Building
State House, Station 34
Augusta, ME 04333
(207) 582-8707
FAX (207) 289-5295

Maryland
501 St. Paul Place
Stanbalt Building, 7th Floor, South
Baltimore, MD 21202
(301) 333-2520
FAX (301) 333-1229

Massachusetts
280 Friend Street
Boston, MA 02114
(617) 727-7189
FAX (617) 727-7189

Michigan
611 West Ottawa Street, 2nd Floor,
  North
P.O. Box 30220
Lansing, MI 48909
(517) 373-9273
FAX (517) 373-7285

Minnesota
500 Metro Square Building, 5th Floor
St. Paul, MN 55101
(612) 296-6848
FAX (612) 296-4328

Mississippi
1804 Walter Sillers Building
P.O. Box 79
Jackson, MS 39205
(601) 359-3569

Missouri
301 West High Street, 6 North
P.O. Box 690
Jefferson City, MO 65102-0690
(314) 751-2451
FAX (314) 751-1165

Montana
126 North Sanders
Mitchell Building, Room 270
P.O. Box 4009
Helena, MT 59601
(406) 444-2040
FAX (406) 444-3497

Nebraska ·
Terminal Building
941 O Street, Suite 400
Lincoln, NE 68508
(402) 471-2201
FAX (402) 471-4610

Nevada
Nye Building
201 South Fall Street
Carson City, NV 89701
(702) 885-4270
FAX (702) 885-4486

New Hampshire
169 Manchester Street
Concord, NH 03301
(603) 271-2261
FAX (603) 224-1427

New Jersey
20 West State Street
Trenton, NJ 08625
(609) 292-5363
FAX (609) 633-3601; (609) 393-5063

New Mexico
PERA Building
P.O. Drawer 1269
Santa Fe, NM 87504-1269
(505) 827-4500

New York
160 West Broadway
New York, NY 10013
(212) 602-0429
NY FAX (212) 602-0437
Albany FAX (518) 473-4600

North Carolina
Dobbs Building
P.O. Box 26387
Raleigh, NC 27611
(919) 733-7343
FAX (919) 733-6495

North Dakota
Capitol Building,
  5th Floor
Bismarck, ND 58505
(701) 224-2440
FAX (701) 224-3000

Ohio
2100 Stella Court
Columbus, OH 43266-0566
(614) 644-2658

Oklahoma
1901 North Walnut
P.O. Box 53408
Oklahoma City, OK 73152-3408
(405) 521-2828
FAX (405) 521-2828

Oregon
21 Labor and Industries Building
Salem, OR 97310
(503) 378-4271

Pennsylvania
Strawberry Square, 13th Floor
Harrisburg, PA 17120
(717) 787-5173
FAX (717) 783-1059

Puerto Rico
Fernandez Juncos Station
P.O. Box 8330
Santurce, PR 00910
(809) 722-8686
FAX (809) 724-5197

Rhode Island
233 Richmond Street, Suite 237
Providence, RI 02903-4237
(401) 277-2246

South Carolina
1612 Marion Street
P.O. Box 100105
Columbia, SC 29202-3105
(803) 737-6117

South Dakota
Insurance Building
910 East Sioux Avenue
Pierre, SD 57501
(605) 773-3563
FAX (605) 773-4840

Tennessee
Volunteer Plaza
500 James Robertson Parkway
Nashville, TN 37219
(615) 741-2241
FAX (615) 741-1583

Texas
1110 San Jacinto Boulevard
Austin, TX 78701-1998
(512) 463-9979
FAX (512) 463-0866

Utah
160 East Third Street
Heber M. Wells Building
P.O. Box 45803
Salt Lake City, UT 84145
(801) 530-6400

Vermont
State Office Building
Montpelier, VT 05602
(802) 828-3301

Virgin Islands
Kongens Gade, No. 18
St. Thomas, Virgin Islands 00802
(809) 774-2991
FAX (809) 774-6953

Virginia
700 Jefferson Building
P.O. Box 1157
Richmond, VA 23209
(804) 786-3741
FAX (804) 786-3396

Washington
Insurance Building, AQ21
Olympia, WA 98504
(206) 753-7301
FAX (206) 586-3535

West Virginia
2019 Washington Street, E
Charleston, WV 25305
(304) 348-3394
FAX (304) 348-0412

Wisconsin
123 West Washington Avenue
P.O. Box 7873
Madison, WI 53707
(608) 266-0102

Wyoming
Herschler Building
122 West 25th Street
Cheyenne, WY 82002
(307) 777-7401
FAX (307) 777-5895

Internal Revenue Service (IRS)
Listed in local phone directories
(800) 554-4477

The IRS has an automated service called Tele-Tax that provides recorded tax information and is tollfree. During the filing season its Tax Counseling for the Elderly provides free assistance to taxpayers who are 60 and older. Taxpayers interested in this service should call the toll-free telephone assistance number listed in the U.S. Government section of local phone directories under Internal Revenue Service and ask for the nearest TCE assistance site available.

Medicare Carriers

The Health Care Financing Administration (HCFA) contracts with insurance companies to oversee the administration of the Medicare program. Bills and inquiries should be sent to the appropriate state carrier listed below.

Alabama
Medicare/Blue Cross–Blue Shield of
   Alabama
P.O. Box C-140
Birmingham, AL 35283
(800) 292-8855; (205) 988-2244

Alaska
Medicare/Aetna Life & Casualty
200 SW Market Street
P.O. Box 1998
Portland, OR 97207-1998
(800) 547-6333

American Samoa
Medicare/Hawaii Medical Services Assn.
818 Keeaumoku
Honolulu, HI 96808
(808) 944-2247

Arizona
Medicare/Aetna Life & Casualty
P.O. Box 37200
Phoenix, AZ 85069
(800) 352-0411; (602) 861-1968

Arkansas
Medicare/Arkansas Blue Cross and Blue
   Shield
A Mutual Insurance Company
P.O. Box 1418
Little Rock, AR 72203
(800) 482-5525; (501) 378-2320

California
*Counties of Los Angeles, Orange, San
   Diego, Ventura, Imperial, San Luis
   Obispo, Santa Barbara:*
Medicare/Transamerica Occidental Life
   Insurance Co.
Box 50061
Upland, CA 91785-0061
(800) 252-9020; (213) 748-2311

Rest of state:
Medicare Claims Department
Blue Shield of California
Chico, CA 95976

In area codes 209, 408, 415, 707, 916:
(800) 952-8627; (916) 743-1583
In area codes 213, 619, 714, 805, 818:
(800) 848-7713; (714) 824-0900

Colorado
Medicare/Blue Shield of Colorado
700 Broadway
Denver, CO 80273
(800) 332-6681; (303) 831-2661

Connecticut
Medicare/The Travelers Ins. Co.
P.O. Box 5005
Wallingford, CT 06493-5005
(800) 982-6819; in Hartford (203)
   728-6783

Delaware
Medicare/Pennsylvania Blue Shield
P.O. Box 65
Camp Hill, PA 17011
(800) 851-3535

District of Columbia
Medicare/Pennsylvania Blue Shield
P.O. Box 100
Camp Hill, PA 17011
(800) 233-1124

Florida
Medicare/Blue Shield of Florida, Inc.
P.O. Box 2525
Jacksonville, FL 32231
(800) 333-7586; (904) 355-3680

Georgia
Aetna Life & Casualty
12052 Middleground Road, Suite A
Savannah, GA 31419
(912) 927-0934

Guam
Medicare/Aetna Life & Casualty
P.O. Box 3947
Honolulu, HI 96812
(808) 524-1240

Hawaii
Medicare/Aetna Life & Casualty
P.O. Box 3947
Honolulu, HI 96812
(800) 272-5242; (808) 524-1240

Idaho
EQUICOR, Inc.
P.O. Box 8048
Boise, ID 83707
(800) 632-6574; (208) 342-7763

Illinois
Medicare Claims
Blue Cross & Blue Shield of Illinois
P.O. Box 4422
Marion, IL 62959
(800) 642-6930; (312) 938-8000

Indiana
Medicare Part B
Associated Ins. Companies, Inc.
P.O. Box 7073
Indianapolis, IN 46207
(800) 622-4792; (317) 842-4151

Iowa
Medicare/Blue Shield of Iowa
636 Grand
Des Moines, IA 50309
(800) 532-1285; (515) 245-4785

Kansas
Counties of Johnson, Wyandotte:
Medicare/Blue Shield of Kansas City
P.O. Box 169
Kansas City, MO 64141
(800) 892-5900; (816) 561-0900

Rest of state:
Medicare/Blue Shield of Kansas
P.O. Box 239
Topeka, KS 66601
(800) 432-3531; (913) 232-3773

Kentucky
Medicare Part B
Blue Cross & Blue Shield of Kentucky
100 East Vine Street
Lexington, KY 40507
(800) 432-9255; (606) 233-1441

Louisiana
Blue Cross & Blue Shield of Louisiana
   Medicare Administration
P.O. Box 95024
Baton Rouge, LA 70895-9024
(800) 462-9666
In New Orleans (504) 529-1494
In Baton Rouge (504) 272-1242

Maine
Medicare/Blue Shield of
   Massachusetts/Tri-State
P.O. Box 1010
Biddeford, ME 04005
(800) 492-0919

Maryland
*Counties of Montgomery, Prince
    Georges:*
Medicare/Pennsylvania Blue Shield
P.O. Box 100
Camp Hill, PA 17011
(800) 233-1124

Rest of state:
Maryland Blue Shield, Inc.
700 East Joppa Road
Towson, MD 21204
(800) 492-4795; (301) 561-4160

Massachusetts
Medicare/Blue Shield of Massachusetts,
    Inc.
55 Accord Park Drive
Rockland, MA 02371
(800) 882-1228

Michigan
Medicare Part B
Michigan Blue Cross & Blue Shield
P.O. Box 2201
Detroit, MI 48231-2201
In area code 313 (800) 482-4045
In area code 517 (800) 322-0607
In area code 616 (800) 442-8020
In area code 906 (800) 562-7802
In Detroit (313) 225-8200

Minnesota
*Counties of Anoka, Dakota, Filmore,
    Goodhue, Hennepin, Houston,
    Olmstead, Ramsey, Wabasha,
    Washington, Winona:*
Medicare/The Travelers Ins. Co.
8120 Penn Avenue
South Bloomington, MN 55431
(800) 352-2762; (612) 884-7171

Rest of state:
Medicare Blue Shield of Minnesota
P.O. Box 64357
St. Paul, MN 55164
(800) 392-0343; (612) 456-5070

Mississippi
Medicare/The Travelers Ins. Co.
P.O. Box 22545
Jackson, MS 39225-2545
(800) 682-5417; (601) 956-0372

Missouri
*Counties of Andrew, Atchison, Bates,
    Benton, Buchanan, Caldwell, Carroll,
    Cass, Clay, Clinton, Davies, DeKalb,
    Gentry, Grundy, Harrison, Henry,
    Holt, Jackson, Johnson, Lafayette,
    Livingston, Mercer, Nodaway, Pettis,
    Platte, Ray, St. Clair, Saline, Vernon,
    Worth:*
Medicare/Blue Shield of Kansas City
P.O. Box 169
Kansas City, MO 64141
(800) 892-5900; (816) 561-0900

Rest of state:
Medicare General American Life
    Insurance Co.
P.O. Box 505
St. Louis, MO 63166
(800) 392-3070; (314) 843-8880

Montana
Medicare/Blue Shield of Montana, Inc.
2501 Beltview
P.O. Box 4310
Helena, MT 59604
(800) 332-6146; (406) 444-8350

Nebraska
See Iowa

Nevada
Medicare/Aetna Life & Casualty
P.O. Box 37230
Phoenix, AZ 85069
(800) 528-0311

New Hampshire
Medicare/Blue Shield of Massachusetts/
  Tri-State
P.O. Box 1010
Biddeford, ME 04005
(800) 447-1142

New Jersey
See Pennsylvania

New Mexico
Medicare/Aetna Life & Casualty
P.O. Box 25500
Oklahoma City, OK 73125-0500
(800) 423-2925
In Albuquerque (505) 843-7771

New York
Counties of Bronx, Kings, New York,
  Richmond:
Medicare/Empire Blue Cross & Blue
  Shield
P.O. Box 100
Yorktown Heights, NY 10598
(212) 490-4444

Counties of Columbia, Delaware,
  Dutchess, Greene, Nassau, Orange,
  Putnam, Rockland, Suffolk, Sullivan,
  Ulster, Westchester:
Medicare/Empire Blue Cross & Blue
  Shield
P.O. Box 100
Yorktown Heights, NY 10598
(800) 442-8430

County of Queens:
Medicare/Group Health, Inc.
P.O. Box A966, Times Square Station
New York, NY 10036
(212) 760-6790

Rest of state:
Medicare
Blue Shield of Western New York
P.O. Box 0600
Binghamton, NY 13902-0600
(800) 252-6550; (607) 772-6906

North Carolina
Equicor Inc., Medicare Administration
1 Tried Center, Suite 240
7736 McCloud Road
Greensboro, NC 27409
(919) 665-0341; (919) 665-0348
(800) 672-3071

North Dakota
Medicare/Blue Shield of North Dakota
4510 13th Avenue, SW
Fargo, ND 58121-0001
(800) 247-2267; (701) 282-1100

Northern Mariana Islands
Medicare/Aetna Life & Casualty
P.O. Box 3947
Honolulu, HI 96812
(808) 524-1240

Ohio
Medicare/Nationwide Mutual Ins. Co.
P.O. Box 57
Columbus, OH 43216
(800) 282-0530; (614) 249-7157

Oklahoma
Medicare/Aetna Life & Casualty
701 NW 63rd Street, Suite 300
Oklahoma City, OK 73116-7693
(800) 522-9079; (405) 848-7711

Oregon
Medicare/Aetna Life & Casualty
200 SW Market Street
P.O. Box 1997
Portland, OR 97207-1997
(800) 452-0125; (503) 222-6831

Pennsylvania
Medicare/Pennsylvania Blue Shield
Box 65
Camp Hill, PA 17011
(800) 382-1274

Puerto Rico
Medicare/Seguros De Servicio De
Salud De Puerto Rico
Call Box 71391
San Juan, PR 00936
(137-800) 462-7385; (809) 759-9191

Rhode Island
Medicare/Blue Shield of Rhode Island
444 Westminster Mall
Providence, RI 02901
(800) 662-5170; (401) 861-2273

South Carolina
Medicare Part B
Blue Cross & Blue Shield of South
    Carolina
Fontaine Road Business Center
300 Arbor Lake Drive, Suite 1300
Columbia, SC 29223
(800) 922-2340; (803) 754-0639

South Dakota
Medicare Part B
Blue Shield of North Dakota
4510 13th Avenue, SW
Fargo, ND 58121-0001
(800) 437-4762

Tennessee
EQUICOR, Inc.
P.O. Box 1465
Nashville, TN 37202
(800) 342-8900; (615) 244-5650

Texas
Medicare/Blue Cross & Blue Shield of
    Texas, Inc.
P.O. Box 660031
Dallas, TX 75266-0031
(800) 442-2620

Utah
Medicare/Blue Shield of Utah
P.O. Box 30269
2455 Parley's Way
Salt Lake City, UT 84130-0269
(800) 426-3477; (801) 481-6196

Vermont
Medicare/Blue Shield of
    Massachusetts/Tri-State
P.O. Box 1010
Biddeford, ME 04005
(800) 447-1142

Virgin Islands
Medicare/Seguros De Servicio De Salud
    De Puerto Rico
Call Box 71391
San Juan, PR 00936
(137-800) 462-2970; (809) 759-9191

Virginia
Counties of Arlington, Fairfax;
cities of Alexandria, Falls Church,
    Fairfax:
Medicare/Pennsylvania Blue Shield
P.O. Box 100
Camp Hill, PA 17011
(800) 233-1124

Rest of state:
Medicare/The Travelers Ins. Co.
P.O. Box 26463
Richmond, VA 23261
(800) 552-3423; (804) 254-4130

Washington
Medicare/Washington Physicians'
    Service
Mail to your local Medical Service
    Bureau. If you do not know which
    bureau handles your claim, mail to:
Medicare Washington Physicians'
    Service
4th and Battery Building, 6th Floor
2401 4th Avenue
Seattle, WA 98121
In King County (800) 422-4087;
    (206) 464-3711
In Spokane (800) 572-5256;
    (509) 536-4550
In Kitsap (800) 552-7114;
    (206) 377-5576
In Pierce (206) 597-6530
Others: Collect if out of call area

West Virginia
Medicare/Nationwide Mutual Insurance
  Co.
P.O. Box 57
Columbus, OH 43216
(800) 848-0106

Wisconsin
Medicare/WPS
Box 1787
Madison, WI 53701
(800) 362-7221
In Madison (608) 221-3330
In Milwaukee (414) 931-1071

Wyoming
EQUICOR, Inc.
P.O. Box 628
102 Indian Hills Shopping Center
Cheyenne, WY 82003
(800) 442-2371; (307) 632-9381

Medicaid Offices

State Medicaid offices are housed in state welfare departments. Older consumers who would like information on Medicaid eligibility and benefits should contact the state agency listed below.

Alabama
Alabama Medicaid Agency
2500 Fairlane Drive
Montgomery, AL 36130
(205) 277-2710
FAX (205) 270-1876

Alaska
Division of Medical Assistance
Department of Health and Social
  Services
P.O. Box H-07
Juneau, AK 99811
(907) 465-3355
FAX (907) 465-3068

Arizona
Arizona Health Care Cost Containment
  System (AHCCCS)
801 East Jefferson
Phoenix, AZ 85034
(602) 234-3655
FAX (602) 258-5943

Arkansas
Office of Long-Term Care
Division of Economic and Medical
  Services
Arkansas Department of Human
  Services
P.O. Box 1437
Little Rock, AR 72203
(501) 682-8487
FAX (501) 682-6571

Office of Medical Services
Division of Economic and Medical
  Services
Arkansas Department of Human
  Services
P.O. Box 1437
Little Rock, AR 72203
(501) 682-8338
FAX (501) 682-6571

Colorado
Bureau of Medical Services
Department of Social Services
1575 Sherman, 6th Floor
Denver, CO 80203
(303) 866-5901

Connecticut
Medical Care Administration
Department of Income Maintenance
110 Bartholomew Avenue
Hartford, CT 06106
(203) 566-2934
FAX (203) 566-6652

Delaware
Medical Services
Department of Health and Social Services
Delaware State Hospital
New Castle, DE 19720
(302) 421-6139

District of Columbia
Office of Health Care Financing
D.C. Department of Human Services
1331 H Street, NW, Suite 500
Washington, DC 20005
(202) 727-0735

Florida
Secretary for Medicaid
Department of Health and
    Rehabilitative Services
1321 Winewood Boulevard
Tallahassee, FL 32399-0700
(904) 488-3560
FAX (904) 487-4272 PX100
FAX (904) 487-2238 (Type 5) UF600SF

Georgia
Georgia Department of Medical
    Assistance
Floyd Veterans Memorial Building
West Tower, 1220C
2 Martin Luther King, Jr., Drive, SE
Atlanta, GA 30334
(404) 656-4479
FAX (404) 651-9496

Guam
Bureau of Health Care Financing
Department of Public Health and
    Social Services
P.O. Box 2816
Agana, Guam 96910
Overseas operator: 734-2944

Hawaii
Health Care Administration Division
Department of Social Services and
    Housing
P.O. Box 339
Honolulu, HI 96809
(808) 548-3855

Idaho
Bureau of Medical Assistance
Department of Health and Welfare
450 West State Street
Statehouse Mail
Boise, ID 83720
(208) 334-5794
FAX (208) 334-5817

Illinois
Division of Medical Programs
Illinois Department of Public Aid
628 East Adams
Springfield, IL 62761
(217) 782-2570

Indiana
Medicaid Director
Indiana State Department of Public
    Welfare
100 North Senate Avenue
State Office Building, Room 702
Indianapolis, IN 46204
(317) 232-4324

Iowa
Bureau of Medical Services
Department of Human Services
Hoover State Office Building, 5th Floor
Des Moines, IA 50319
(515) 281-8794
FAX (515) 281-4597

Kansas
Medical Services Division
Department of Social and Rehabilitation
   Services
State Office Building
Topeka, KS 66612
(913) 296-3981
FAX (913) 296-1158

Kentucky
Department of Medicaid Services
Cabinet for Human Resources
275 East Main Street
Frankfort, KY 40621
(502) 564-6535
FAX (502) 564-3232

Louisiana
Medical Assistance Division
Department of Health and Human
   Resources
P.O. Box 94065
Baton Rouge, LA 70804
(504) 342-3956

Maine
Bureau of Medical Services
Department of Human Services
State House Station, No. 11
Augusta, ME 04333
(207) 289-2674
FAX (207) 626-5555

Maryland
Department of Health and Mental
   Hygiene
201 West Preston Street
Baltimore, MD 21201
(301) 225-6535

Massachusetts
Associate Commissioner for Medical
   Payments
Department of Public Welfare
180 Tremont Street
Boston, MA 02111
(617) 574-0205

Michigan
Medical Services Administration
Department of Social Services
921 West Holmes
P.O. Box 30037
Lansing, MI 48909
(517) 334-7262

Minnesota
Health Care and Residential Programs
Department of Human Services
P.O. Box 43170
St. Paul, MN 55164
(612) 296-2766
FAX (612) 297-1539

Mississippi
Division of Medicaid
Office of the Governor
Robert E. Lee Building, Room 801
239 North Lamar Street
Jackson, MS 39201-1311
(601) 359-6050
FAX (601) 359-6089

Missouri
Division of Medical Services
Department of Social Services
P.O. Box 6500
Jefferson City, MO 65102
(314) 751-6922
FAX (314) 751-3203

Montana
Economic Assistance Division
Department of Social and Rehabilitation
   Services
P.O. Box 4210
Helena, MT 59604
(406) 444-4540
FAX (406) 444-1970

Nebraska
Medical Services Division
Department of Social Services
301 Centennial Mall South, 5th Floor
Lincoln, NE 68509
(402) 471-9330
FAX (402) 471-9449

Nevada
Nevada Medicaid Welfare Division
Department of Human Resources
Capitol Complex
2527 North Carson Street
Carson City, NV 89710
(702) 885-4698
FAX (702) 885-4733

New Hampshire
Office of Medical Services
New Hampshire Division of Human
 Services
Department of Health and Human
 Services
6 Hazen Drive
Concord, NH 03301-6521
(603) 271-4353
FAX (603) 271-2896

New Jersey
Division of Medical Assistance and
 Health Services
Department of Human Services
CN-712 Quakerbridge Plaza
Trenton, NJ 08625
(609) 588-2602
FAX (609) 588-3583

New Mexico
Medical Assistance Division
Department of Human Services
P.O. Box 2348
Santa Fe, NM 87503-2348
(505) 827-4315
FAX (505) 827-4191

New York
Division of Medical Assistance
State Department of Social Services
Ten Eyck Office Building
40 North Pearl Street
Albany, NY 12243
(518) 474-9132

North Carolina
Division of Medical Assistance
Department of Human Resources
1985 Umstead Drive
Raleigh, NC 27603
(919) 733-2060

North Dakota
Medical Services
North Dakota Department of Human
 Services
State Capitol Building
Bismarck, ND 58505
(701) 224-2321
FAX (701) 224-3000

Northern Mariana Islands
Department of Public Health and
 Environmental Services
Commonwealth of the Northern
 Mariana Islands
Saipan, CM 96950
(670) 234-8950, ext. 2905

Ohio
Medicaid Administration
Department of Human Services
30 East Broad Street, 31st Floor
Columbus, OH 43266-0423
(614) 466-3196
FAX (614) 466-8493

Oklahoma
Division of Medical Services
Department of Human Services
P.O. Box 25352
Oklahoma City, OK 73125
(405) 557-2539
FAX (405) 521-8816

Oregon
Department of Human Resources
313 Public Service Building
Salem, OR 97310
(503) 378-4728
FAX (503) 378-6432

Health Services Section
Adult and Family Services Division
Department of Human Resources
203 Public Service Building
Salem, OR 97310
(503) 378-2263
FAX (503) 378-8404

Pennsylvania
Department of Public Welfare
Room 515
Health and Welfare Building
Harrisburg, PA 17120
(717) 787-1870
FAX (717) 787-4639

Puerto Rico
Health Economy Office
Department of Health
P.O. Box 9342
San Juan, PR 00936
(809) 765-9941

Rhode Island
Division of Medical Services
Department of Human Services
Aime J. Forand Building
600 New London Avenue
Cranston, RI 02920
(401) 464-3575
FAX (401) 464-1876

South Carolina
Director for Program Operation
Health and Human Services Finance
   Commission
P.O. Box 8206
Columbia, SC 29202
(803) 253-6100

South Dakota
Medical Services
Department of Social Services
Kneip Building
701 North Illinois Street
Pierre, SD 57501
(605) 773-3495
FAX (605) 773-4855

Tennessee
Bureau of Medicaid
Department of Health and Environment
729 Church Street
Nashville, TN 37219
(615) 741-0213

Texas
Health Care Services
Texas Department of Human Services
P.O. Box 2960, Main Code 600-W
Austin, TX 78769
(512) 450-3050
FAX (512) 450-4176; (512) 450-3017

Services to the Aged and Disabled
Department of Human Services
P.O. Box 2960
Austin, TX 78769
(512) 450-3192

Utah
Division of Health Care Financing
Utah Department of Health
P.O. Box 16580
Salt Lake City, UT 84116-0580
(801) 538-6151

Vermont
Division of Medicaid
Department of Social Welfare
Vermont Agency of Human Services
103 South Main Street
Waterbury, VT 05676
(802) 241-2880

Virgin Islands
Bureau of Health Insurance and Medical
  Assistance
Department of Health
P.O. Box 7309
Government of the Virgin Islands
Charlotte Amalie, St. Thomas 00801
(809) 774-4624; (809) 773-2150

Virginia
Virginia Department of Medical
  Assistance Services
600 East Broad Street, Suite 1300
Richmond, VA 23219
(804) 786-7933
FAX (804) 225-4512

Washington
Division of Medical Assistance
Department of Social and Health
  Services
Mail Stop HB-41
Olympia, WA 98504
(206) 753-1777
FAX (206) 753-9152

West Virginia
Bureau of Medical Care
West Virginia Department of Human
  Services
1900 Washington Street East
Charleston, WV 25305
(304) 348-8990

Wisconsin
Bureau of Health Care Financing
  Division of Health
Wisconsin Department of Health and
  Social Services
1 West Wilson Street, Room 244
P.O. Box 309
Madison, WI 53701
(608) 266-2522

Wyoming
Medical Assistance State Program
Department of Health and Social
  Services
448 Hathaway Building
Cheyenne, WY 82002
(307) 777-7531

Peer Review Organizations (PROs)

Peer Review Organizations are groups of doctors and other professionals who are under contract with the HCFA to review the services provided by hospitals and skilled-nursing facilities, to make sure that the services meet professional standards and are as economical as possible. Among other things, appeals for Medicare reimbursement of hospital stays must be made to local PROs. The following is a list of state Peer Review Organizations.

Alabama
Alabama Quality Assurance Foundation
236 Goodwin Crest Drive,
Twin Towers East Building, Suite 300
Birmingham, AL 35209
(205) 942-0785

Alaska
Professional Review Organization for
  Washington
10700 Meridian Avenue North,
  Suite 300
Seattle, WA 98133
(206) 364-9700

American Samoa/Guam
Hawaii Medical Services Association
818 Keeaumoku Street
P.O. Box 860
Honolulu, HI 96808
(808) 944-3581

Arizona
Health Services Advisory Group, Inc.
301 East Bethany Home Road
Building B, Suite 157
Phoenix, AZ 85012
(602) 264-6382

Arkansas
Arkansas Foundation for Medical Care,
    Inc.
P.O. Box 1508
809 Garrison Avenue
Fort Smith, AR 72902
(501) 785-2471

California
California Medical Review Inc.
1388 Sutter Street, Suite 1100
San Francisco, CA 94109
(415) 923-2000

Colorado
Colorado Foundation for Medical Care
Building 2, Suite 400
6825 East Tennessee Avenue
Denver, CO 80224
(303) 321-8642

Connecticut
Connecticut Peer Review Organization,
    Inc.
384 Pratt Street
Meriden, CT 06450
(203) 237-2773

Delaware
West Virginia Medical Institute, Inc.
3412 Chesterfield Avenue, SE
Charleston, WV 25304
(304) 925-0461

District of Columbia
Delmarva Foundation for Medical Care,
    Inc.
341 B North Aurora Street
Easton, MD 21601
(301) 822-0697

Florida
Professional Foundation for Health Care
    Inc.
2907 Bay to Bay Boulevard, Suite 100
Tampa, FL 33629
(813) 831-6273

Georgia
Georgia Medical Care Foundation
4 Executive Park Drive, NE, Suite 1300
Atlanta, GA 30329
(404) 982-0411

Hawaii
Hawaii Medical Services Association
818 Keeaumoku Street
P.O. Box 860
Honolulu, HI 96808
(808) 944-3586

Idaho
Professional Review Organization for
    Washington
10700 Meridian Avenue North, Suite
    300
Seattle, WA 98133
(206) 364-9700

Illinois
Crescent Counties Foundation for
    Medical Care
350 Shuman Boulevard, Suite 240
Naperville, IL 60540
(312) 357-8770

Indiana
Indiana Peer Review, Inc.
501 Congressional Boulevard, Suite 300
Carmel, IN 46032
(317) 573-6888

Iowa
Iowa Foundation for Medical Care
Colony Park
3737 Woodland Avenue, Suite 500
West Des Moines, IA 50265
(515) 223-2900

Kansas
The Kansas Foundation for Medical
  Care, Inc.
2947 SW Wanamaker Drive
Topeka, KS 66614
(913) 273-2552

Kentucky
Kentucky Peer Review, Inc.
10300 Linn Station Road, Suite 100
Louisville, KY 40223
(502) 429-0995

Louisiana
Louisiana Health Care Review
9357 Interline Avenue, Suite 200
Baton Rouge, LA 70809
(504) 926-6353

Maine
Health Care Review, Inc.
The Weld Building
345 Blackstone Boulevard
Providence, RI 02906
(401) 331-6661

Maryland
Delmarva Foundation for Medical Care,
  Inc.
341 B North Aurora Street
Easton, MD 21601
(301) 822-0697

Massachusetts
Massachusetts Peer Review
  Organization, Inc.
300 Bearhill Road
Waltham, MA 02154
(617) 890-0011

Michigan
Michigan Peer Review Organization
40500 Ann Arbor Road, Suite 200
Plymouth, MI 48170
(313) 459-0900

Minnesota
Foundation for Health Care Evaluation
One Appletree Square, Suite 700
Minneapolis, MN 55420
(612) 854-3306

Mississippi
Mississippi Foundation for Medical
  Care, Inc.
P.O. Box 4665
1900 North West Street
Jackson, MS 39216
(601) 948-8894

Missouri
Missouri Patient Care Review
  Foundation
311 Ellis Boulevard, Suite A
Jefferson City, MO 65101
(314) 634-4441

Montana
Montana-Wyoming Foundation for
  Medical Care
P.O. Box 5117
21 North Main
Helena, MT 59604
(406) 443-4020

Nebraska
Iowa Foundation for Medical Care (NE)
Colony Park Building, Suite 500
3737 Woodland Avenue
West Des Moines, IA 50265
(515) 223-2900

Nevada
Nevada Physicians Review Organization
4600 Kietzke Lane
Building A, Suite 108
Reno, NV 89502
(702) 826-1996

New Hampshire
New Hampshire Foundation for
   Medical Care
P.O. Box 578
110 Locust Street
Dover, NH 03820
(603) 749-1641

New Jersey
The Peer Review Organization of New
   Jersey, Inc.
Central Division
Brier Hill Court, Building J
East Brunswick, NJ 08816
(201) 238-5570

New Mexico
New Mexico Medical Review
   Association
707 Broadway, NE, Suite 200
P.O. Box 9900
Albuquerque, NM 87119
(505) 842-6236

New York
Empire State Medical Scientific and
   Educational Foundation, Inc.
420 Lakeview Road
Box 5434
Lake Success, NY 11042
(516) 437-8134

North Carolina
Medical Review of North Carolina
P.O. Box 37309
1011 Schaub Drive, Suite 200
Raleigh, NC 27627
(919) 851-2955

North Dakota
North Dakota Health Care Review, Inc.
900 North Broadway, Suite 212
Minot, ND 58701
(701) 852-4231

Ohio
Peer Review Systems, Inc.
3700 Corporate Drive, Suite 250
Columbus, OH 43229
(614) 895-9900

Oklahoma
Oklahoma Foundation for Peer Review,
   Inc.
5801 Broadway Extension
The Paragon Building, Suite 400
Oklahoma City, OK 73118
(405) 840-2891

Oregon
Oregon Medical Professional Review
   Organization
Suite 300
1220 Southwest Morrison
Portland, OR 97205
(503) 243-1151

Pennsylvania
Keystone Peer Review Organization,
   Inc.
645 North 12th Street
P.O. Box 618
Lemoyne, PA 17043
(717) 975-9600

Puerto Rico
Puerto Rico Foundation for Medical
   Care
Mercantile Plaza, Suite 605
Hato Rey, PR 00918
(809) 753-6705

Rhode Island
Health Care Review, Inc.
The Weld Building
345 Blackstone Boulevard
Providence, RI 02906
(401) 331-6661

South Carolina
Metrolina Medical Foundation/South
    Carolina PRO
1000 Carolina Commerce Center
1642 West Highway 160
Fort Mill, SC 29715
(803) 548-8400

South Dakota
South Dakota Foundation for Medical
    Care
1323 South Minnesota Avenue
Sioux Falls, SD 57105
(605) 336-3505

Tennessee
Mid-South Foundation for Medical Care
6401 Poplar Avenue, Suite 400
Memphis, TN 38119
(901) 682-0381

Texas
Texas Medical Foundation
Barton Oaks Plaza Two, Suite 200
901 Mopac Expressway South
Austin, TX 78746
(512) 329-6610

Utah
Utah Professional Standard Review
    Organization
540 East 5th South Street, Suite 200
Salt Lake City, UT 84102
(801) 532-7545

Vermont
New Hampshire Foundation for
    Medical Care
P.O. Box 578
110 Locust Street
Dover, NH 03820
(603) 749-1641

Virgin Islands
Virgin Islands Medical Institute
P.O. Box 1556
Christiansted
St.Croix, Virgin Islands 00820
(809) 778-6470

Virginia
Medical Society of Virginia Review
    Organization
1904 Byrd Avenue, Room 120
P.O. Box 6569
Richmond, VA 23230
(804) 289-5320

Washington
Professional Review Organization for
    Washington
10700 Meridian Avenue North, Suite
    300
Seattle, WA 98133
(206) 364-9700

West Virginia
West Virginia Medical Institute, Inc.
3412 Chesterfield Avenue, SE
Charleston, WV 25304
(304) 925-0461

Wisconsin
Wisconsin Peer Review Organization
2001 West Beltline Highway
Madison, WI 53713
(608) 274-1940

Wyoming
Montana-Wyoming Foundation for
    Medical Care
P.O. Box 5117
21 North Main
Helena, MT 59604
(406) 443-4020

U.S. House of Representatives, Select Committee on Aging
Congressman Edward Roybal (D-CA), Chairman
712 Rayburn House Office Building, Annex 1
Washington, DC 20515
(202) 226-3375

> The House Select Committee on Aging is a congressional oversight committee serving as the focus in the Congress for information on programs and policies affecting the elderly. It is responsible for informing and advising members of Congress, conducting congressional oversight of federal agencies and programs for older Americans, and making a full study and investigation of the various concerns of the aged that come to its attention. The committee also publishes materials of importance to the elderly. For example, a recent report analyzed out-of-pocket health-care costs for Medicare beneficiaries. The committee publishes *Aging Notes,* a monthly that describes committee activities.

U.S. Senate, Special Committee on Aging
Senator David Pryor (D-AK), Chairman
SDG-41
Washington, DC 20510
(202) 224-5364

> The committee is responsible for studying all issues that affect older people and reporting its findings to Congress. It investigates such issues as Medicare, Medicaid, HMOs, and supplemental health insurance. The committee also conducts oversight on all federal programs that affect the elderly. It publishes a number of committee prints of interest to older health consumers, including *Developments in Aging,* a two-volume annual report to Congress that analyzes the major events of the previous year of interest to the elderly. The committee staff are available for answering requests for information on programs affecting the elderly.

Health, Social Service, and Long-Term-Care Organizations

American Association of Homes for the Aging (AAHA)
Sheldon Goldberg, President
1129 Twentieth Street, NW, Suite 400
Washington, DC 20036
(202) 296-5960

AAHA is a highly effective association representing the community-based, nonprofit nursing homes in the United States as well as independent housing programs, continuing-care retirement communities, and community-service programs. The association publishes updated consumer materials for the public such as two informative pamphlets on how to select nursing homes and continuing-care retirement communities. AAHA's state associations, listed below, are valuable resources for locating nursing homes, community services, and continuing-care retirement communities.

Alabama Association of Homes for the Aging
Mr. Wray Tomlin, President
c/o Methodist Homes for Aging
1424 Montclair Road
Birmingham, AL 35210
(205) 956-4150

Arizona Association of Homes for the Aging
Ms. Randi Weiss, Executive Director
204 Abacus Tower
3030 North Third Street
Phoenix, AZ 85012
(602) 264-1984

California Association of Homes for the Aging
Mr. Dean R. Shetler, President
7311 Greenhaven Drive, Suite 175
Sacramento, CA 95831
(916) 392-5111

Colorado Association of Homes & Services for the Aging
Mr. John Torres, Executive Director
2140 South Holly Street
Denver, CO 80222
(303) 759-8688

Connecticut Association of Non-Profit Facilities for the Aged
Ms. Rosalind Berman, President
110 Barnes Road
P.O. Box 90
Wallingford, CT 06492
(203) 269-7443

Florida Association of Homes for the Aging
Ms. Karen Torgesen, Executive Director
1018 Thomasville Road, Suite 200Y
Tallahassee, FL 32303-6236
(904) 222-3562

Georgia Association of Homes &
  Services for the Aging
Ms. Vickie Moody-Beasley, President
2719 Buford Highway, Suite 213
Atlanta, GA 30324
(404) 728-0223

Illinois Association of Homes for the
  Aging
Mr. Dennis R. Bozzi, Executive Director
911 North Elm Street, Suite 228
Hinsdale, IL 60521
(708) 325-6170
FAX (708) 325-0749

Indiana Association of Homes for the
  Aging
Mr. George F. Heighway, Executive
  Director
1265 West 86th Street
Indianapolis, IN 46260
(317) 257-1115

Iowa Association of Homes for the
  Aging
Ms. Judi Pierick, Executive Director
4685 Merle Hay Road, Suite 101
Des Moines, IA 50322
(515) 270-1198

Kansas Association of Homes for the
  Aging
Mr. John Grace, President
641 S.W. Harrison Street
Topeka, KS 66603
(913) 233-7443

Kentucky Association of Homes for the
  Aging
Ms. Louise Schroader, Executive Director
1244 South Fourth Street
Louisville, KY 40203
(502) 635-6468

Louisiana Association of Homes &
  Services for the Aging
Ms. Allison Gremillon, Executive
  Director
2431 South Acadian Thruway, Suite 280
Baton Rouge, LA 70808
(504) 928-6894

Maryland Association of Nonprofit
  Homes for the Aging
Ms. Ann M. MacKay, President
6263 Bright Plume
Columbia, MD 21044-3749
(301) 740-4585
FAX (301) 290-5285 (cover sheet must
  include Ann's name and phone
  number)

National Capital Area Assn. of Homes
  for the Aging
Mr. David Zwald, President Pro Tem
c/o Ginger Cove
4000 River Crescent Drive
Annapolis, MD 21401
(301) 266-7300

Association of Massachusetts Homes for
  the Aging
Mr. Merlin Southwick, Executive
  Director
45 Bromfield Street
Boston, MA 02108
(617) 423-0718

Michigan Nonprofit Homes Association,
  Inc.
Mr. Donald J. Bentsen, Executive
  Director
1615 East Kalamazoo Street
Lansing, MI 48912
(517) 372-7540

Minnesota Association of Homes for the
  Aging
Ms. Gayle Kvenvold, President & CEO
2221 University Avenue, S.E., Suite 425
Minneapolis, MN 55414
(612) 331-5571

Missouri Association of Homes for the
  Aging
Mr. James Nagel, President
6925 Hampton Avenue
St. Louis, MO 63109-3902
(314) 353-9050
FAX (314) 353-4771

Montana Association of Homes for the
  Aging
Ms. Jean Johnson, Executive Director
34 West Sixth Street, 2E
P.O. Box 5774
Helena, MT 59601
(406) 443-1185

Nebraska Association of Homes for the
  Aging
Mr. Ron Jensen, Executive Director
1320 Lincoln Mall, Suite 9
Lincoln, NE 68508
(402) 477-7015

Northern New England Association of
  Homes and Services for the Aging
Ms. Christine C. Hallock, President
c/o Hunt Community
10 Allds Street
Nashua, NH 03060
(603) 882-6511

New Jersey Association of Nonprofit
  Homes for the Aging
Ms. Karen J. Uebele, Executive Director
760 Alexander Road, CN #1
Princeton, NJ 08540
(609) 452-1161
FAX (609) 452-2907

New York Association of Homes &
  Services for the Aging
Mr. Carl Young, President
194 Washington Avenue, 4th Floor
Albany, NY 12210
(518) 449-2707
FAX (518) 455-8908

Rochester Area Association of Homes &
  Services for the Aging
Ms. Nancy Newton, Executive Director
259 Monroe Avenue
Rochester, NY 14607
(716) 454-7300

North Carolina Association of Nonprofit
  Homes for the Aging
Ms. Sarah R. Shaber, Executive Director
1717 Park Drive
Raleigh, NC 27605
(919) 821-0803

North Dakota Nursing Home
  Association
Mr. Robert Howe, Senior Vice President
Kirkwood Office Tower
919 Arbor Avenue
Bismarck, ND 58501
(701) 224-9440

Association of Ohio Philanthropic
  Homes and Housing for the Aging
Mr. Clark R. Law, Executive Director
36 West Gay Street
Columbus, OH 43215
(614) 221-2882
FAX (614) 221-4490

Oregon Association of Homes for the
  Aging
Ms. Sally P. Goodwin, Executive Director
7150 South West Hampton Street,
  Suite 206
Tigard, OR 97223
(503) 684-3788

Pennsylvania Association of Nonprofit
   Homes for the Aging
Rev. David J. Keller, Executive Director
P.O. Box 698
3425 Simpson Ferry Road
Camp Hill, PA 17011
(717) 763-5724
FAX (717) 763-1057

Rhode Island Association of Facilities
   for the Aged
Ms. Sheila Sousa, President
St. Antoine Residence
400 Menden Road
North Smithfield, RI 02895
(401) 767-3500

South Carolina Association of Nonprofit
   Homes for the Aging
Ms. Joan V. Young, President
c/o Presbyterian Home of South
   Carolina
Highway 56 North
Clinton, SC 29325
(803) 833-5190

South Dakota Association of Homes for
   the Aging
Ms. Betsy Reck, Executive Director
330 North Main Avenue, Suite 201
P.O. Box 639
Sioux Falls, SD 57101
(605) 338-6621
FAX (605) 338-0770

Tennessee Association of Homes for the
   Aging
Ms. Jennifer Humphreys, Executive
   Director
1305 Rolling Meadow Court
Mt. Juliet, TN 37122
(615) 758-7440

Texas Association of Homes for the Aging
Ms. Sandy Derrow, President
720 Brazos Street, Suite 1104
Austin, TX 78701
(512) 477-6994

Virginia Association of Nonprofit
   Homes for the Aging
Ms. Ann McGee, President
4900 Augusta Avenue, Suite 104
Richmond, VA 23230
(804) 353-8141

Washington Association of Homes for
   the Aging
Ms. Karen L. Tynes, Executive Director
444 N.E. Ravenna Boulevard, Suite 109
Seattle, WA 98115
(206) 526-8450

Wisconsin Association of Homes &
   Services for the Aging
Mr. John Sauer, Executive Director
6400 Gisholt Drive, Suite 203
Madison, WI 53713
(608) 222-5086

AAHA Regional Directors

Ms. Leslie A. Knight
Director, Midwest Region
American Association of Homes for the
   Aging
911 North Elm Street, Suite 228
Hinsdale, IL 60521
(708) 323-6755
FAX (708) 325-0749

Ms. Mary M. Reilly
Director, Western Region
American Association of Homes for the
   Aging
5010 Aspen Drive
Littleton, CO 80123
(303) 795-5465

Ms. Anne Brooks
Executive Director, Northeast Region
American Association of Homes for the
   Aging
2001 Jefferson Court
Ambler, PA 19002
(215) 628-2232

Canadian Associations

Ontario Association of Non-Profit
   Homes and Services for Seniors
Mr. Michael J. Klejman, Executive
   Director
7 Director Court, Suite 102
Woodbridge, Ontario, Canada L4L 4Z5
(416) 851-8821

Association des Centres D'Accuiel du
   Quebec
Mr. Michel Clair, Director General
1001 de Maisonneuve Est #1100
Montreal, Quebec, Canada H2L 4P9
(514) 597-1007

Saskatchewan Association of Special
   Care Homes
Mr. Bun Wasiuta, Executive Director
2-1540 Albert/Regina
Saskatchewan, Canada S4P 2S4
(306) 565-0744

American Health Care Association (AHCA)
Paul R. Willging, Executive Vice-President
1201 L Street, NW
Washington, DC 20005
(202) 842-8444

The American Health Care Association and its state affiliates
represent licensed nursing homes and related long-term-care
facilities. The majority of AHCA member facilities are propri-
etary. AHCA state affiliates, listed below, have information on
the member facilities providing services in local areas.

Alabama
Alabama Nursing Home Association
4156 Carmichael Road
Montgomery, AL 36106
(205) 271-6214

Alaska
Health Association of Alaska
319 Seward Street
Juneau, AK 99801
(907) 586-1790

Arizona
Arizona Nursing Home Association
1817 North Third Street, Suite 200
Phoenix, AZ 85004
(602) 258-8996

Arkansas
Arkansas Long Term Care Assn.
1324 West Capitol Avenue
Little Rock, AR 72201
(501) 374-4422

California
California Assn. of Health Facs.
1251 Beacon Boulevard
West Sacramento, CA 95691-3461
(916) 371-4700

Colorado
Colorado Health Care Association
1600 Sherman Street, Suite 420
Denver, CO 80203
(303) 861-8228

Connecticut
Connecticut Association of Health Care
   Facilities
131 New London Turnpike, Suite 18
Glastonbury, CT 06033
(203) 659-0391

Delaware
Delaware Health Care Facilities
   Association
3801 Kennett Pike
Building D-200
P.O. Box 4420
Wilmington, DE 19807
(302) 656-7864

District of Columbia
District of Columbia Health Care
   Association
11312 Old Club Road
Rockville, MD 20852-4537
(301) 881-4113

Florida
Florida Health Care Association
307 West Park
P.O. Box 1459
Tallahassee, FL 32302-1459
(904) 224-3907

Georgia
Georgia Health Care Association
3735 Memorial Drive
P.O. Box 36349
Decatur, GA 30032
(404) 284-8700

Hawaii
Healthcare Association of Hawaii
932 Ward Avenue, Suite 430
Honolulu, HI 96814
(808) 521-8961

Idaho
Idaho Health Care Association
830 West Washington, No. 206
Box 2623
Boise, ID 83701
(208) 343-9735

Illinois
Illinois Health Care Association
1029 South 4th Street
Springfield, IL 62703
(217) 528-6455

Indiana
Indiana Health Care Association
One North Capitol, Suite 1115
Indianapolis, IN 46204
(317) 636-6406

Iowa
Iowa Health Care Association
950 Twelfth Street
Des Moines, IA 50309
(515) 282-0666

Kansas
Kansas Health Care Association
221 Southwest 33rd
Topeka, KS 66611
(913) 267-6003

Kentucky
Kentucky Association of Health Care
   Facilities
P.O. Box 692
903 Collins Lane
Frankfort, KY 40602 (40601)
(502) 875-1500

Louisiana
Louisiana Health Care Association
7921 Picardy Avenue
Baton Rouge, LA 70809
(504) 769-3705

Maine
Maine Health Care Association
303 State Street
Augusta, ME 04330
(207) 623-1146

Maryland
Health Facilities Association of Maryland
229 Hanover Street
Annapolis, MD 21401
(301) 269-1390
(301) 261-1416 from DC only

Massachusetts
Massachusetts Federation of Nursing
    Homes, Inc.
990 Washington Street, Suite 207
Dedham, MA 02026
(507) 835-2800

Michigan
Health Care Association of Michigan
7413 Westshire Drive
Lansing, MI 48917
(517) 627-1561

Minnesota
Care Providers of Minnesota
2850 Metro Drive, Suite 200
Minneapolis, MN 55425
(612) 854-2844

Mississippi
Mississippi Health Care Association
4444 North State Street
Jackson, MS 39206
(601) 362-2527

Missouri
Missouri Health Care Association
236 Metro Drive
Jefferson City, MO 65101
(314) 893-2060

Montana
Montana Health Care Association
36 South Last Chance Gulch, Suite A
Helena, MT 59601
(406) 443-2876

Nebraska
Nebraska Health Care Association
3100 "O" Street, Suite 7
Lincoln, NE 68510
(402) 435-3551

Nevada
Nevada Health Care Association
1150 East Williams, Suite 203
Box 3226
Carson City, NV 89702
(702) 885-1006

New Hampshire
New Hampshire Health Care Association
125 Airport Road
Concord, NH 03301
(603) 225-0900

New Jersey
New Jersey Association/Health Care
    Facilities
2131 Route 33
Lexington Square Commons
Trenton, NJ 08690
(609) 890-8700

New Mexico
New Mexico Health Care Association
1024 Eubank, NE, Suite D
Albuquerque, NM 87112
(505) 296-0021

New York
New York State Health Facilities
    Association
111 Washington Avenue, Suite 700
Albany, NY 12210-2213
(518) 462-4800

North Carolina
North Carolina Health Care Facilities
    Association
5109 Bur Oak Circle
Raleigh, NC 27612
(919) 782-3827

North Dakota
North Dakota Health Care Association
1600 East Interstate Avenue, Suite 9
Bismarck, ND 58501
(701) 222-0660

Ohio
Ohio Health Care Association
50 Northwoods Boulevard
Worthington, OH 43235
(614) 436-4154

Oregon
Oregon Health Care Association
12200 North Jantzen Avenue, Suite 380
Portland, OR 97217
(503) 285-9600

Pennsylvania
Pennsylvania Health Care Association
2400 Park Drive
Harrisburg, PA 17110
(717) 657-4902

Rhode Island
Rhode Island Health Care Association
144 Bignall Street
Warwick, RI 02888
(401) 785-9530

South Carolina
South Carolina Health Care Association
1706 Senate Street
Columbia, SC 29201
(803) 256-2681

South Dakota
South Dakota Health Care Association
804 North Western Avenue
Sioux Falls, SD 57104-2098
(605) 339-2071

Tennessee
Tennessee Health Care Association
P.O. Box 100129-2809
Foster Avenue
Nashville, TN 37210
(615) 834-6520

Texas
Texas Health Care Association
4214 Medical Parkway, 3rd Floor
Austin, TX 78756
(512) 458-1257

Utah
Utah Health Care Association
1255 East 3900 South
Salt Lake City, UT 84124
(801) 268-9622

Vermont
Vermont Health Care Association
58 East State Street
Montpelier, VT 05602
(802) 229-5700

Virginia
Virginia Health Care Association
2112 West Laburnum Avenue, Suite 206
Richmond, VA 23227
(804) 353-9101

Washington
Washington Health Care Association
2120 State Avenue, NE, Suite 102
Olympia, WA 98506
(206) 352-3304

West Virginia
West Virginia Health Care Association
1115 Quarrier Street
Charleston, WV 25301
(304) 346-4575 or 346-4576

Wisconsin
Wisconsin Association of Nursing Homes
14 South Carroll Street, Suite 200
Madison, WI 53703-3376
(608) 257-0125

Wyoming
Wyoming Health Care Association
P.O. Box 2186
809 Silver Sage Avenue
Cheyenne, WY 82003
(307) 635-2175

Foundation for Hospice and Homecare (FHH)
William J. Halamandaris, Chief Executive Officer
519 C Street, NE
Washington, DC 20002
(202) 547-5263

> FHH promotes high standards of patient care for hospice and
> home health care services. The foundation accredits homemaker–
> home health aide agencies, conducts research, and provides
> technical assistance to agencies. In 1987 FHH absorbed the
> National Homecaring Council (NHC), formerly the National
> Council for Homemaker Services, and the National Council for
> Homemaker–Home Health Aide Services. NHC now functions
> as a division of the foundation.

Group Health Association of America (GHAA)
Susan Pisano, Public Relations Associate
1129 Twentieth Street, NW, No. 600
Washington, DC 20036
(202) 778-3200

> GHAA is a membership organization representing the HMO
> industry. With 225 member plans representing 60 percent of
> all HMOs, the association played a key role in assuring the
> elderly the right to get their care in an HMO. GHAA's library is
> the most extensive collection on prepaid, managed care. GHAA
> conducts a yearly survey of HMOs that provides a database for
> comparing plans.

Home Health Care Associations

> State home health agencies represent and monitor the quality of
> agencies within individual states. Older consumers who would
> like information on home health care within their state should
> contact the state association listed below.

Alabama
Alabama Association of Home
    Health Agencies
2368 Fairlane Drive, Suite E-37
Montgomery, AL 36116
(205) 272-3538

Alaska
Alaska Home Care Association
44539 Sterling Highway
Soldotna, AK 99699
(907) 262-4750

Arizona
Arizona Association for Home Care
P.O. Box 36794
Phoenix, AZ 85067
(602) 955-0262

Arkansas
Arkansas Association for Home Health
  Agencies
1501 N. University, Suite 400
Little Rock, AR 72207
(501) 664-7870

California
California Association for Health
  Services at Home
660 J Street, Suite 290
Sacramento, CA 95814
(916) 443-8055

Colorado
Colorado Association of Home Health
  Agencies
7600 East Arapahoe Road, Suite 316
Englewood, CO 80112
(303) 694-4728

Connecticut
Connecticut Association for Home Care,
  Inc.
110 Barnes Road
P.O. Box 90
Wallingford, CT 06492
(203) 265-9931

Delaware
Delaware Association of Home Health
  Services
Route 3, Box 15
Berlin, MD 21811
(301) 749-2202

District of Columbia
Capitol Home Health Association
P.O. Box 70407
Washington, DC 20088
(202) 293-2193

Florida
Florida Association of Home Health
  Agencies, Inc.
110 South Monroe Street, Suite 200
Tallahassee, FL 32301
(904) 224-4226

Georgia
Georgia Association of Home Health
  Agencies, Inc.
6666 Powers Ferry Road, Suite 260
Atlanta, GA 30339
(404) 984-9704

Hawaii
The Hawaii Association for Home Care
Ala Moana Building, Suite 1320
1441 Kapiolani Boulevard
Honolulu, HI 96814
(808) 955-1102

Idaho
Idaho Association of Home Health
  Agencies
200 North 4th Street, Suite 20
Boise, ID 83702-6001
(208) 345-0500

Illinois
Illinois Council of Home Health Services
2008 Dempster Street
Evanston, IL 60202
(312) 328-6654

Indiana
Indiana Association of Home Health
  Agencies
8888 Keystone Crossing, Suite 1000
Indianapolis, IN 46240
(317) 844-6630

Iowa
Iowa Association of Home Health
  Agencies
Homeward
902 Ridgewood
Ames, IA 50010
(515) 239-2314

Kansas
Kansas Home Care Association
4101 West 13th Street
Lawrence, KS 66046
(913) 841-2833

Kentucky
Kentucky Home Health Association
153 Patchen Drive, Suite 40
Lexington, KY 40502
(606) 268-2574

Louisiana
Hospital HomeCare Association
of Louisiana
P.O. Box 80720
Baton Rouge, LA 70898-0720
(504) 928-0026

Louisiana Association of HHA
10985 North Harrell's Ferry Road,
Suite E
Baton Rouge, LA 70816
(504) 275-1791

Maine
Home Care Alliance of Maine
One Park Drive
Rockland, ME 04841
(207) 594-9561

Maryland
Maryland Association for Home Care,
Inc.
5820 Southwestern Boulevard
Baltimore, MD 21227
(301) 242-1973

Massachusetts
Massachusetts Association of
Community Health Agencies
100 Boylston Street, Suite 724
Boston, MA 02116
(617) 482-8830

Massachusetts Council for Homemaker–
Home Health Aide Services
34¹/₂ Beacon Street
Boston, MA 02108
(617) 523-6400

Visiting Nurses Associations of
Massachusetts
900 Providence Highway RR
Dedham, MA 02026
(617) 326-9996

Michigan
Michigan Home Health Assembly
4990 Northwind Drive, Suite 220
East Lansing, MI 48823
(517) 332-1195
FAX (517) 332-1196

Minnesota
MLN Assembly of Home Health
2353 North Rice Street, Suite 220
St. Paul, MN 55113
(612) 481-1277

Mississippi
Mississippi Home Health Association
3103 Bridge Port Lane
Madison, MS 39110
(601) 856-9161

Mississippi Hospital Association
Society for Home Care
P.O. Box 16958
Hattiesburg, MS 39404
(601) 288-4344

Missouri
Missouri Alliance for Home Care
1233 Jefferson
Jefferson City, MO 65101
(314) 634-7772

Missouri Council for Homemaker Services
204 West Rollins Street
Moberly, MO 65270
(816) 263-1517

Montana
Montana Association of HHA
Courthouse, Room 308
P.O. Box 35033
Billings, MT 59107
(406) 256-2757

Nebraska
Nebraska Association of Home and
   Community Health Agencies
P.O. Box 95007
Lincoln, NE 68509
(402) 471-2771

Nevada
Home Health Care Association of
   Nevada
P.O. Box 20188
Reno, NV 89515
(702) 853-2155

New Hampshire
Home Care Association of New
   Hampshire
117 Manchester Street
Concord, NH 03301
(603) 225-5597

New Jersey
Home Care Council of New Jersey
60 South Fullerton Avenue
Montclair, NJ 07042
(201) 744-5524

Home Health Agency Assembly of New
   Jersey, Inc.
760 Alexander Road, CN-1
Princeton, NJ 08543-0001
(609) 452-8855

New Mexico
New Mexico Association for Home Care
Route 9, Box 90 M
Santa Fe, NM 87505
(505) 988-1186

New York
Home Care Association of New York
   State, Inc.
840 James Street
Syracuse, NY 13203
(315) 475-7229

New York State Association of Health
   Care Providers, Inc.
90 State Street, Suite 909
Albany, NY 12207
(518) 463-1118

North Carolina
North Carolina Association for Home
   Care, Inc.
1005 Dresser Court
Raleigh, NC 27609
(919) 878-0500

North Dakota
North Dakota Association of Home
   Health Agencies
212 North 4th Street
Green Tree Square
Bismarck, ND 58501
(701) 223-1385

Ohio
Ohio Council of Home Health Agencies
5008 Pine Creek Drive, Suite B
Westerville, OH 43081-4899
(614) 898-7684

Ohio Council of Homemaker–Home
   Health Aide Services, Inc.
500 Hanna Building
1422 Euclid Avenue
Cleveland, OH 44115-1989
(216) 621-7201

Oklahoma
Home Health–Home Care Association
   of Oklahoma
P.O. Box 76351
Oklahoma City, OK 73147
(405) 942-4660

Oregon
Oregon Association for Home Care
Box 510
Salem, OR 97308
(503) 399-7517

Pennsylvania
Pennsylvania Association of HHA
2400 Park Drive
Harrisburg, PA 17110
(717) 657-7605

Puerto Rico
Puerto Rico Home Health Agencies
    Association
677 Bernardette, Urb Loudes
Trujillo Alto, PR 00760
(809) 726-0960

Rhode Island
Association of Home Health Agencies of
    Rhode Island, Inc.
142 Kenyon Avenue
Wakefield, RI 02879
(401) 789-0232

Coalition of VNA's of Rhode Island
P.O. Box 3026
Providence, RI 02906
(401) 737-6050

South Carolina
South Carolina Home Care Association
P.O. Box 767
Irmo, SC 29063
(803) 781-0926

South Dakota
South Dakota Home Health Association
P.O. Box 942
Watertown, SD 57102
(605) 341-7118

Tennessee
Tennessee Association for Home Health
226 Capitol Boulevard, Suite 510
Nashville, TN 37219
(615) 254-3333

Texas
Texas Association of HHA
One La Costa Office Building
1016 La Posada Drive, Suite 129
Austin, TX 78752
(512) 459-4303

Utah
Utah Association of Home Health
    Agencies
1058 East 900 South
Salt Lake City, UT 84105
(801) 322-3430

Vermont
Vermont Assembly of Home Health
    Agencies
52 State Street
Montpelier, VT 05602
(802) 229-0579

Virginia
Virginia Association for Home Care
Koger Executive Center
1501 Santa Rosa Road, Suite B-12
Richmond, VA 23288
(804) 285-8636

Washington
Home Care Association of Washington
406 Main Street, Suite 116
Edmonds, WA 98020
(206) 775-8120

West Virginia
West Virginia Council of Home Health
    Agencies, Inc.
3137 Pennsylvania Avenue, Suite B
Weirton, WV 26062
(304) 723-2730

Wisconsin
Wisconsin Homecare Organization
6441 Enterprise Lane
Madison, WI 53719
(608) 274-8118

Joint Commission on Accreditation of Healthcare Organizations (JCAHO)
875 North Michigan Avenue, Suite 2201
Chicago, IL 60611
(312) 642-6061

> Formerly the Joint Commission on Accreditation of Hospitals, JCAHO offers voluntary accreditation, education, and consultation services to a variety of health-care organizations, including nursing homes, hospitals, and home health care organizations. Recent publications include the *Long-Term Care Standards Manual*.

National Association of Area Agencies on Aging (N4A)
John Linkous, Executive Director
600 Maryland Avenue, SW, Suite West 208
Washington, DC 20024
(202) 484-7520

> N4A represents and provides assistance to the 660-plus Area Agencies on Aging (AAAs) in the country, which are funded under the Older Americans Act. AAAs fund local services to older adults on a non–means-tested basis. However, services are in great demand and waiting lists are long. N4A publishes a list of their members as well as public-information materials about Older Americans Act programs.

National Association of State Units on Aging (NASUA)
Daniel Quirk, Executive Director
2033 K Street, NW, Suite 304
Washington, DC 20006
(202) 785-0707

> NASUA is a membership association of the State Units on Aging, which are funded under the Older Americans Act. NASUA staff members serve as a voice on the state perspective on aging at a national level and provide training and assistance to state units. Older consumers who would like information on community services for the aging available on a state level should contact their state unit listed below.

Alabama
Commission on Aging
Second Floor
136 Catoma Street
Montgomery, AL 36130
(205) 261-5743

Alaska
Older Alaskans Commission
Department of Administration
Pouch C-Mail Station 0209
Juneau, AK 99811-0209
(907) 465-3250

Arizona
Aging and Adult Administration
Department of Economic Security
1400 West Washington Street
Phoenix, AZ 85007
(602) 255-4446

Arkansas
Division of Aging and Adult Servs.
Arkansas Department of Human
  Services
1417 Donaghey Plaza South
7th and Main Streets
Little Rock, AR 72201
(501) 682-2441

California
Department of Aging
1600 K Street
Sacramento, CA 95814
(916) 322-5290

Colorado
Aging and Adult Services
Department of Social Services
1575 Sherman Street, 10th Floor
Denver, CO 80203-1714
(303) 866-5931

Connecticut
Department on Aging
175 Main Street
Hartford, CT 06106
(203) 566-3238

Delaware
Division on Aging
Department of Health and Social
  Services
1901 North DuPont Highway
New Castle, DE 19720
(302) 421-6791

District of Columbia
Office on Aging
1424 K Street, NW, 2nd Floor
Washington, DC 20005
(202) 724-5626

Florida
Program Office of Aging and Adult Services
Department of Health and Rehabilitative
  Services
1317 Winewood Boulevard
Tallahassee, FL 32301
(904) 488-8922

Georgia
Office of Aging
878 Peachtree Street, NE, Room 632
Atlanta, GA 30309
(404) 894-5333

Guam
Division of Senior Citizens
Department of Public Health & Social
  Services
Government of Guam
P.O. Box 2816
Agana, Guam 96910

Hawaii
Executive Office on Aging
Office of the Governor
335 Merchant Street, Room 241
Honolulu, HI 96813
(808) 548-2593

Idaho
Office on Aging
Room 114—Statehouse
Boise, ID 83720
(208) 334-3833

Illinois
Department on Aging
421 East Capitol Avenue
Springfield, IL 62701
(217) 785-2870

Indiana
Division of Aging Services
Department of Human Services
251 North Illinois Street
P.O. Box 7083
Indianapolis, IN 46207-7083
(317) 232-7020

Iowa
Department of Elder Affairs
Suite 236, Jewett Building
914 Grand Avenue
Des Moines, IA 50319
(515) 281-5187

Kansas
Department on Aging
Docking State Office Building, 122-S
915 S.W. Harrison
Topeka, KS 66612-1500
(913) 296-4986

Kentucky
Division of Aging Services
Cabinet for Human Resources
CHR Building—6th West
275 East Main Street
Frankfort, KY 40621
(502) 564-6930

Louisiana
Office of Elderly Affairs
P.O. Box 80374
Baton Rouge, LA 70898
(504) 925-1700

Maine
Bureau of Maine's Elderly
Department of Human Services
State House—Station 11
Augusta, ME 04333
(207) 289-2561

Maryland
Office on Aging
State Office Building
301 West Preston Street, Room 1004
Baltimore, MD 21201
(301) 225-1100

Massachusetts
Executive Office of Elder Affairs
38 Chauncy Street
Boston, MA 02111
(617) 727-7750

Michigan
Office of Services to the Aging
P.O. Box 30026
Lansing, MI 48909
(517) 373-8230

Minnesota
Board on Aging
4th Floor, Human Services Building
444 Lafayette Road
St. Paul, MN 55155-3843
(612) 296-2770

Mississippi
Council on Aging
301 West Pearl Street
Jackson, MS 39203-3092
(601) 949-2070

Missouri
Division on Aging
Department of Social Services
P.O. Box 1337
2701 West Main Street
Jefferson City, MO 65102
(314) 751-3082

Montana
Department of Family Services
48 North Last Chance Gulch
P.O. Box 8005
Helena, MT 59604
(406) 444-5900

Nebraska
Department on Aging
P.O. Box 95044
301 Centennial Mall—South
Lincoln, NE 68509
(402) 471-2306

Nevada
Division for Aging Services
Department of Human Resources
340 North 11th Street
Las Vegas, NV 89101
(702) 486-3545

New Hampshire
Div. of Elderly and Adult Servs.
6 Hazen Drive
Concord, NH 03301-6501
(603) 271-4680

New Jersey
Division on Aging
Department of Community Affairs,
  CN807
South Broad and Front Streets
Trenton, NJ 08625-0807
(609) 292-4833

New Mexico
State Agency on Aging
224 East Palace Avenue—4th Floor
La Villa Rivera Building
Santa Fe, NM 87501
(505) 827-7640

New York
Office for the Aging
New York State Plaza
Agency Building 2
Albany, NY 12223
(518) 474-4425

North Carolina
Division of Aging
1985 Umstead Drive, Kirby Bldg.
Raleigh, NC 27603
(919) 733-3983

North Dakota
Aging Services
Department of Human Services
State Capitol Building
Bismarck, ND 58505
(701) 224-2577

Northern Mariana Islands
Office of Aging
Department of Community and Cultural
  Affairs
Civic Center—Susupe
Saipan, Northern Mariana Islands
96950
Tel. Nos. 9411 or 9732

Ohio
Department of Aging
50 West Broad Street—9th Floor
Columbus, OH 43266-0501
(614) 466-5500

Oklahoma
Aging Services Division
Department of Human Services
P.O. Box 25352
Oklahoma City, OK 73125
(405) 521-2281

Oregon
Senior Services Division
313 Public Service Building
Salem, OR 97310
(503) 378-4728

Pennsylvania
Department of Aging
231 State Street
Harrisburg, PA 17101-1195
(717) 783-1550

Puerto Rico
Gericulture Commission
Department of Social Services
Apartado 11398
Santurce, PR 00910
(809) 721-4010

Rhode Island
Department of Elderly Affairs
79 Washington Street
Providence, RI 02903
(401) 277-2858

(American) Samoa
Territorial Administration on Aging
Office of the Governor
Pago Pago, American Samoa 96799
011 (684) 633-1252

South Carolina
Commission on Aging
400 Arbor Lake Drive, Suite B-500
Columbia, SC 29223
(803) 735-0210

South Dakota
Office of Adult Services and Aging
700 North Illinois Street
Kneip Building
Pierre, SD 57501
(605) 773-3656

Tennessee
Commission on Aging
706 Church Street, Suite 201
Nashville, TN 37219-5573
(615) 741-2056

Texas
Department on Aging
P.O. Box 12786, Capitol Station
1949 IH 35, South
Austin, TX 78741-3702
(512) 444-2727

Trust Territory of the Pacific
Office of Elderly Programs
Community Development Division
Government of TTPI
Saipan, Mariana Islands 96950
Tel. Nos. 9335 or 9336

Utah
Division of Aging and Adult Services
Department of Social Services
120 North—200 West
Box 45500
Salt Lake City, UT 84145-0500
(801) 538-3910

Vermont
Office on Aging
103 South Main Street
Waterbury, VT 05676
(802) 241-2400

Virgin Islands
Department of Human Services
6F Havensight Mall—Charlotte Amalie
St. Thomas, Virgin Islands 00801
(809) 774-5884

Virginia
Department for the Aging
700 Centre, 10th Floor
700 East Franklin Street
Richmond, VA 23219-2327
(804) 225-2271

Washington
Aging and Adult Services
    Administration
Department of Social and Health
    Services
OB-44A
Olympia, WA 98504
(206) 586-3768

West Virginia
Commission on Aging
Holly Grove—State Capitol
Charleston, WV 25305
(304) 348-3317

Wisconsin
Bureau of Aging
Division of Community Services
One West Wilson Street, Room 480
Madison, WI 53702
(608) 266-2536

Wyoming
Commission on Aging
Hathaway Building—Room 139
Cheyenne, WY 82002-0710
(307) 777-7986

National Homecaring Council (NHC)
William Halamandaris, Chief Executive Officer
519 C Street, NE
Stanton Park
Washington, DC 20002
(202) 547-6586

> NHC is a division of the Foundation for Hospice and Home Care. The council conducts a consumer-education program, promotes development of standards, administers an agency-accreditation program, and sponsors conferences. NHC publishes the *Directory of Accredited/Approved Homemaker–Home Health Aide Services* annually. It also publishes *HomeCare News* biweekly in conjunction with the National Association for Home Care.

National Hospice Association (NHA)
John J. Mahoney, President
1901 North Moore Street, Suite 901
Arlington, VA 22209
(703) 243-5900

> The National Hospice Association promotes standards of care in program planning and implementation and monitors health-care legislation and regulation affecting hospice care. The association operates a telephone referral service on hospice programs throughout the country. NHA publishes a *Guide to the Nation's Hospices* and a journal and newsletter for members.

National Institute of Senior Centers (NISC)
Jean M. Coyle, Coordinator
c/o National Council on the Aging
West Wing 100
600 Maryland Avenue, SW
Washington, DC 20024
(202) 479-1200

> NISC's 1,600 members are individuals or organizations affiliated with senior centers at the local, state, or national level. The institute assists senior centers, organizations, and communities in developing new centers and upgrading established ones. It develops standards for centers nationwide. NISC publishes a quarterly newsletter, the *Senior Center Report.*

National Institute on Adult Daycare (NIAD)
c/o National Council on the Aging
Dorothy K. Howe, Coordinator
600 Maryland Avenue, SW, West Wing 100
Washington, DC 20024
(202) 479-1200

> NIAD's 1,200 members are adult-day-care practitioners, health and social-service planners, and individuals involved in planning and providing services to older persons. The institute furnishes training and technical assistance for day-care personnel, develops standards and guidelines for programs, and surveys adult day-care regulations and legislation. It publishes the *Adult Day Care Quarterly,* a newsletter reporting on adult day-care centers and general aging issues.

Health and Social Service Professional Organizations

Aging Network Services (ANS)
Grace Lebow and Barbara Kane, Co-Directors
Topaz House, Suite 907
4400 East-West Highway
Bethesda, MD 20814
(301) 657-4329

> ANS currently has members across the country who provide quality geriatric assessment services. In some cases health insurance will pay for their services.

American Association for Continuity of Care (AACC)
Sharon Dobson, Coordinator
1101 Connecticut Avenue, NW, Suite 700
Washington, DC 20036
(202) 857-1194

> AACC is an association of health-care professionals including discharge planners, social workers, hospital administrators, and home-care providers. AACC develops and supports legislation on Medicare changes and home health care. The association's membership directory is published annually.

American Public Welfare Association (APWA)
A. Sydney Johnson III, Executive Director
810 First Avenue, NE, Suite 500
Washington, DC 20002
(202) 682-0100

> APWA is a nonprofit association of 10,000 members represent-
> ing state human-service departments, local welfare agencies, and
> social-welfare professionals. Services include the Medicaid Man-
> agement Institute for state Medicaid administrators. The State
> Medicaid Directors' Association is an affiliate of APWA.

Catholic Charities U.S.A. (CCUSA)
Thomas Harvey, Executive Director
1319 F Street, NW, Fourth Floor
Washington, DC 20004
(202) 639-8400

> CCUSA is the central organization for the 633 Catholic Charities
> social-service agencies in the United States. CCUSA maintains a
> consultation and information service and publishes the annual
> *Directory of Diocesan Agencies of Catholic Charities in the U.S.,
> Puerto Rico and Canada.*

Family Service America (FSA)
Geneva B. Johnson, Chief Executive Officer and President
11700 West Lake Park Drive
Milwaukee, WI 53224
(414) 359-2111

> Family Service America is a federation of social-service agencies
> in more than 200 communities providing counseling and other
> services to families. FSA's *Directory of Member Agencies* is
> updated every year.

National Association for Home Care (NAHC)
Val J. Halamandaris, President
519 C Street, NE
Washington, DC 20002
(202) 547-7424

> NAHC is a membership organization of 6,000 home health care
> providers. Its major goal is the promotion of home health care as
> the solution to long-term care. Two of NAHC's current priorities

are adoption of a federal long-term-care policy and expansion of Medicare home health benefits. The association makes a number of publications available to its members, as well as public-information materials for consumers shopping for home health care services. A *National Home Care Directory* will be available in 1990.

National Association of Private Geriatric Care Managers
Rona Bartlestone, President
P.O. Box 6920
Yorkville Station
New York, NY 10128
(212) 316-1111

The National Association of Private Geriatric Care Managers establishes educational and experience requirements for its members, who are specialists in private practice. The names of geriatric care managers are available from the association.

National Association of Social Workers (NASW)
Myark G. Battle, Executive Director
7981 Eastern Avenue
Silver Spring, MD 20910
(301) 565-0333

NASW is the largest association of social workers in the world. The association sets standards for members, develops policy analyses, and publishes basic reference works for members. Its *Social Work Directory* is a guide to locating social workers nationwide.

National Eye Care Project (NECP)
Anna Zammataro, Manager
P.O. Box 6988
San Francisco, CA 94101-6988
(800) 222-EYES

The National Eye Care Project offers medical care to the disadvantaged elderly at no out-of-pocket costs. The project is sponsored by the American Academy of Ophthalmology and is available to persons 65 and older who are U.S. citizens and legal residents. Interested health consumers must not be under the care of an ophthalmologist and must not have seen an ophthalmologist in five years. After calling the 800 number, the individual will be mailed the name of a volunteer ophthalmologist who will treat him or her regardless of ability to pay. The program does not pay for hospital charges, eyeglasses, or prescription drugs.

National Federation of Licensed Practical Nurses (NFLPN)
David C. Kesterson, Interim Executive Director
P.O. Box 18088
Durham, NC 27703
(919) 781-4791

NFLPN is the federation of state associations of licensed practical and vocational nurses. The federation acts as a clearinghouse on practical nursing and aims to improve standards of practice.

National League for Nursing (NLN)
Pamela Maraldo, Executive Officer
Ten Columbus Circle
New York, NY 10019
(212) 582-1022

NLN's 20,000 members include nurses, other health professionals, nursing agencies, nursing educational institutions, departments of nursing in hospitals, and home and community health agencies. The league nationally accredits community health agencies. NLN also collects and disseminates data on nursing services and nursing education and publishes an extensive list of materials for health professionals.

Visiting Nurse Associations of America (VNAA)
Kay Brown, Vice-President
1391 North Speer Boulevard, No. 802
P.O. Box 4637
Denver, CO 80204
(800) 426-2547; in Colorado (303) 629-8622

The VNAA is the organization of the highly regarded Visiting Nurse Associations (VNAs). The VNAs are voluntary, nonprofit home health care agencies, of which there presently are more than 500 nationwide. The association publishes *The Directory of Visiting Nurse Associations in the United States,* which is available for $100 to nonmembers.

Self-Help Organizations

Alzheimer's Association
(formerly the Alzheimer's Disease and Related Disorders Association)
Edward F. Truschke, President
70 East Lake Street
Chicago, IL 60601-5997
(800) 621-0379; in Illinois (800) 572-6037

> The Alzheimer's Association sponsors more than 200 chapters that provide support groups and other services for family members of persons with dementia. The association operates a toll-free hotline, listed above, that will provide information on chapters and programs across the country. AA publishes a quarterly newsletter, brochures, and a handbook of interest to family members.

Children of Aging Parents (CAPS)
Mirca Liberti, Co-Executive Director
2761 Trenton Road
Levittown, PA 19056
(215) 945-6900

> CAPS is a self-help group devoted to helping care givers of the elderly. Although most of CAPS's activities are focused in Pennsylvania and New Jersey, the organization offers advice to interested groups across the country. CAPS publishes a bimonthly newsletter on concerns of older persons and their families, as well as *How To Start a Self-Help Group for Caregivers*.

The Self-Help Center
1600 Dodge Avenue, Suite S-122
Evanston, IL 60201
(312) 328-0470 (24-hour line)

> Although the Self-Help Center is set up specifically to help residents of Illinois locate self-help groups, it also publishes a directory of support-group clearinghouses nationwide. Anyone calling can get the name, address, and phone number of the closest self-help clearinghouse. The directory may be purchased by mailing a check to the above address ($18 by mail in 1989).

Self-Help Clearinghouse
Edward J. Madara, Director
Saint Clares–Riverside Medical Center
Denville, NJ 07834
(201) 625-9565
TDD (201) 625-9053
In New Jersey (800) 367-6274

The Self-Help Clearinghouse has a national database listing more than 600 national and model self-help groups dealing with a wide range of addictions, disabilities, chronic illnesses, bereavement, and other stressful life situations. A new edition of the organization's *Self-Help Source Book,* based on the database, is to be available in 1990.

The following is a list of self-help clearinghouses across the country (clearinghouses are not presently available in every state).

National information/Directories
National Self-Help Clearinghouse
City Univ. of N.Y. Graduate Center,
    Room 1206A
33 West 42nd Street
New York, NY 10036
(212) 840-1259

Self-Help Clearinghouse
Saint Clares–Riverside Medical Center
Denville, NJ 07834
(201) 625-9565; TDD (201) 625-9053

Self-Help Center
1600 Dodge Avenue, Suite S-122
Evanston, IL 60201
(312) 328-0470

Arizona
Rainy Day People Project
P.O. Box 472
Scottsdale, AZ 85252

California
California Self-Help Center
U.C.L.A. Psychology Department
405 Hilgard Avenue
Los Angeles, CA 90024
(213) 825-1799; (800) 222-LINK (in
CA only)

Northern Region Self-Help Center
Mental Health Association
5370 Elvas Avenue, Suite B
Sacramento, CA 95819
(916) 456-2070

Central Valley Self-Help Center
Mental Health Association
P.O. Box 343
Merced, CA 95341
(209) 723-8861

Southern Region Self-Help Center
Mental Health Association of San Diego
3958 Third Avenue
San Diego, CA 92103

Bay Area Self-Help Center
Mental Health Association
2398 Pine Street
San Francisco, CA 94115
(415) 921-4401

Self-Help Clearinghouse of Yolo County
Mental Health Association
P.O. Box 447
Davis, CA 95617
(916) 756-8181

Connecticut
Connecticut Self-Help/Mutual Support
    Network
Consultation Center
19 Howe Street
New Haven, CT 06511
(203) 789-7645

**District of Columbia, Northern Virginia,
    Southern Maryland**
Self-Help Clearinghouse of Greater
    Washington
Mental Health Association of Northern
    Virginia
100 North Washington Street, Suite 232
Falls Church, VA 22046
(703) 536-4100

Illinois
Self-Help Center
1600 Dodge Avenue, Suite S-122
Evanston, IL 60201
(312) 328-0470; (800) 322-MASH (in
    IL only)

Self-Help Center
Family Service of Champaign County
405 South State Street
Champaign, IL 61820
(217) 352-0092

Iowa
Iowa Self-Help Clearinghouse
Iowa Pilot Parents, Inc.
33 North 12th Street
Fort Dodge, IA 50501
(515) 576-5870; (800) 383-4777 (in IA
    only)

Kansas
Self-Help Network
Campus Box 34
Wichita State University
Wichita, KS 67208-1595
(316) 689-3170

Massachusetts
Massachusetts Clearinghouse of Mutual
    Help Groups
Massachusetts Cooperative Extension
113 Skinner Hall
University of Massachusetts
Amherst, MA 01003
(413) 545-2313

Michigan
Michigan Self-Help Clearinghouse
Michigan Protection and Advocacy
    Service
109 West Michigan Avenue, Suite 900
Lansing, MI 48933
(517) 484-7373; (800) 752-5858 (in MI
    only)

Center for Self-Help
Riverwood Center
1485 Highway, M-139
Benton Harbor, MI 49022
(616) 925-0594

Minnesota
Minnesota Mutual Help Resource
    Center
Wilder Foundation Community Care
    Unit
919 Lafond Avenue
St. Paul, MN 55104
(612) 642-4060

Missouri
Support Group Clearinghouse
Kansas City Association for Mental Health
1020 East 63rd Street
Kansas City, MO 64110
(816) 561-HELP

Nebraska
Self-Help Information Services
1601 Euclid Avenue
Lincoln, NE 68502
(402) 476-9668

New Jersey
New Jersey Self-Help Clearinghouse
St. Clares—Riverside Medical Center
Denville, NJ 07834
(201) 625-9565; TDD (201) 625-9053
In NJ (800) FOR-MASH

New York
Brooklyn Self-Help Clearinghouse
Heights Hills Mental Health Service
30 Third Avenue
Brooklyn, NY 11217
(718) 834-7341; (718) 834-7332

Long Island Self-Help Clearinghouse
New York Institute of Technology
Central Islip Campus
Central Islip, NY 11722
(516) 348-3030

New York City Self-Help Clearinghouse,
   Inc.
P.O. Box 022812
Brooklyn, NY 11202
(718) 596-6000

New York State Self-Help Clearinghouse
N.Y. Council on Children & Families
Empire State Plaza, Tower 2
Albany, NY 12224
(518) 474-6293
Maintains listing of additional local
   county self-help clearinghouses
   throughout upstate New York area.

Westchester Self-Help Clearinghouse
Westchester Community College
Academics Arts Building
75 Grasslands Road
Valhalla, NY 10595
(914) 347-3620

Oregon
N.W. Regional Self-Help Clearinghouse
718 West Burnside Street
Portland, OR 97209
(503) 222-5555; (503) 226-9360

Pennsylvania
Self-Help Group Network of the
   Pittsburgh Area
710½ South Avenue
Wilkensburg, PA 15221
(412) 247-5400

S.H.I.N.E. (Self-Help Information
   Network Exchange)
c/o Voluntary Action Center
225 North Washington Avenue
Park Plaza, Lower Level
Scranton, PA 18503
(717) 961-1234

Rhode Island
Support Group Helpline
Rhode Island Department of Health
Cannon Building
Davis Street
Providence, RI 02908

South Carolina
Midland Area Support Group Network
Lexington Medical Center
2720 Sunset Boulevard
West Columbia, SC 29169
(803) 791-9227

Tennessee
Support Group Clearinghouse
Mental Health Association of Knox County
6712 Kingston Pike, No. 203
Knoxville, TN 37919
(614) 584-6736

Texas
Texas Self-Help Clearinghouse
Mental Health Association in Texas
1111 West 24th Street
Austin, TX 78705
(512) 454-3706

Dallas Self-Help Clearinghouse
Mental Health Association of Dallas
   County
2500 Maple Avenue
Dallas, TX 75201-1998
(214) 871-2420

Self-Help Clearinghouse
Mental Health Association in Houston
   & Harris County
2211 Norfolk, Suite 810
Houston, TX 77098
(713) 523-8963

Greater San Antonio Self-Help
   Clearinghouse
Mental Health in Greater San Antonio
1407 North Main
San Antonio, TX 78212
(512) 222-1571

Tarrant County Self-Help Clearinghouse
Mental Health Association of Tarrant
   County
3136 West 4th Street
Fort Worth, TX 76107-2113
(817) 335-5405

Vermont
Vermont Self-Help Clearinghouse
c/o Parents Assistance Line
103 South Main Street
Waterbury, VT 05676
(802) 241-2249; in VT (800) 442-5356

State Health-Insurance Counseling Programs

California

Health Insurance Counseling and Advocacy Program (HICAP)
Department of Aging
1600 K Street
Sacramento, CA 95814

> HICAP is a support network of local volunteers who offer
> health-insurance and Medicare-counseling services to seniors.
> The program is administered by the California Department of
> Aging and is designed to assist persons 60 years of age and older.
> Local projects include community education, individual counsel-
> ing, and advocacy of Medicare-beneficiary interests.

Colorado

Medical Insurance Assistance, Inc. (MIA)
1440 North Hancock
P.O. Box 9634
Colorado Springs, CO 80932

MIA is a private nonprofit corporation assisting senior citizens who need help with Medicare and Medicaid supplemental coverages. Claims are submitted for clients, and follow-up assistance is provided to assure that benefits are paid correctly. MIA provides clients with evaluations and explanations of insurance policies for a better understanding of what insurance will pay and what will have to be paid by the individual. The organization does not charge for its services, but tax-deductible donations are requested.

Retired Senior Volunteer Program (RSVP)
1215 Cedar Street
Boulder, CO 80304

RSVP is a group of volunteers trained by the Health Care Financing Administration (HCFA) and Social Security to assist individuals in dealing with problems with Medicare, Medicaid, and Medicare supplemental insurance. Volunteers are knowledgeable in auto insurance as well as health insurance. A helpful hint sheet is available to provide information on Medicare and other health insurance. Forms with information on how to buy medigap insurance are offered, along with advice on how to steer clear of areas of liability.

Senior Health Insurance Counseling Program (SHIC-P)
P.O. Box 18221
Denver, CO 80210
(303) 333-3482

SHIC-P provides trained volunteer counselors to help older adults understand their Medicare benefits. Services include help with organizing medical bills and recordkeeping, filing insurance claims, and analyzing and comparing Medicare supplemental health insurance, health maintenance organizations, and other options for supplementing Medicare. Volunteers provide services at sites throughout the community and make home visits to those physically unable to reach a counseling site. Bilingual counselors are available. SHIC-P also offers educational programs to many community groups interested in learning about Medicare and related health-insurance issues.

Connecticut

Center for Medicare Advocacy
791 Main Street
Willimantic, CT 06226
(800) 262-4414

> Staffed by attorneys and paralegals, the center provides legal advice, self-help materials, and representation to older adults who are having problems with their Medicare coverage. Legal representation is free to many and on a graduated fee for those who can afford to pay.

Legal Assistance to Medicare Patients (LAMP)
P.O. Box 258
Willimantic, CT 06226

> Like the center described above, LAMP has attorneys who will assist low-income persons who have problems with their Medicare benefits.

Illinois

Senior Health Insurance Program (SHIP)
State of Illinois
Department of Insurance
Springfield, IL 62767

> SHIP is a training and support program for volunteers around the state who provide health-insurance counseling to seniors. Funding is supplied by the state department of insurance.

Massachusetts

Serving Health Information Needs of Elders (SHINE)
Commonwealth of Massachusetts
38 Chauncy Street
Boston, MA 02111

> SHINE is sponsored by the Massachusetts Executive Office of Elder Affairs in conjunction with the Massachusetts Councils on Aging. It provides seniors with information on health insurance

and health-care options. SHINE has developed a network of volunteer counselors to advise seniors, a free service.

Missouri

CLAIM, Community Leaders Assisting the Insured of Missouri

CLAIM is a network of volunteers throughout Missouri who channel complaints and inquiries to the Missouri Division of Insurance. University extension programs work with the division of insurance in establishing and promoting the program. One of CLAIM's three major purposes is to help residents, particularly seniors, to understand the basics of insurance so they can better protect themselves against insurance fraud.

New Jersey

Senior Health Insurance Program (SHIP)
Division of Consumer Protection and Enforcement
State of New Jersey
Department of Insurance
20 West State Street, CN 325
Trenton, NJ 08625

SHIP is a statewide program of trained senior-citizen volunteers available on a one-to-one basis to assist seniors in filing insurance claims and evaluating and comparing insurance policies. The volunteers also help with health-insurance-related questions.

North Carolina

Senior Health Insurance Information Program (SHIP)
North Carolina Department of Insurance
430 North Salisbury Street
Raleigh, NC 27611

SHIP is a statewide program of trained volunteers who assist older adults with health-insurance problems. SHIP has developed a training manual for use in training volunteers.

Washington

Senior Health Insurance Benefits Advisors (SHIBA)
State of Washington
Office of Insurance Commissioner
Olympia Office Insurance Building
Olympia, WA 98504-0321

> SHIBA volunteers answer questions and refer individuals to the proper government agencies where solutions can be found for health insurance problems. Volunteers have been through 25 or more hours of training in the basics of insurance, Medicare, Medicare supplemental insurance, and long-term-care insurance.

Wisconsin

Medigap Hotline
(800) 242-1060

> Wisconsin's medigap hotline is a statewide toll-free number sponsored by the Wisconsin Board on Aging and Long Term Care to answer questions about health insurance and other health-care benefits for the elderly.

Chapter 11

Reference Material

Books

American Association of Retired Persons. *How To Plan Your Successful Retirement*. Glenview, IL: Scott-Foresman and Co., 1989. 128p. $9.95. ISBN 0-673-24889-5.

> AARP's retirement-planning guide contains brief but useful sections on choosing health-care providers, health-care options such as HMOs and IPAs, and tips for keeping down health-care costs.

Altman, Maya, Stuart P. Hanson, and Sherry Almond. *How Do I Pay for My Long-Term Health Care?* Oakland, CA: Berkeley Planning Associates, 1988. 106p. $12.95. ISBN 0-9620825-0-3.

> With funding from the government, Berkeley Planning Associates has developed a useful guide to long-term care and the limitations of Medicare benefits, plus information regarding Medicaid. Although *How Do I Pay for Long-Term Care?* includes silly cartoons that present negative images of aging, the authors present an objective, important view of long-term care. They provide readers help with analyzing policies so that they may choose the best possible long-term-care coverage. Presented in an easy-to-read format, the guide contains useful information for individuals and organizations offering assistance to older persons and their families.

Berko, Robert L. *Consumer's Guide to Social Security Benefits Including Medicare*. South Orange, NJ: Consumer Education Resource Center, 1987. 140p. $9. ISBN 0-934873-04-6.

While the focus of Robert Berko's guide is on the Social Security program, it includes brief but helpful sections on such topics as how to fill out a Medicare claim, where to send Medicare claims, appeals rights, supplemental health insurance, and hospice benefits.

Bloom, Jill. *The Revolution in Health Care HMOs*. Tucson, AZ: The Body Press, 1987. 277p. $9.95. ISBN 0-89586-557-2.

The Revolution in Health Care HMOs is a comprehensive guide to HMOs and their advantages as health-care alternatives. The guide is not written for an older audience; however, it provides excellent background information on this quickly changing industry. A directory of HMOs with telephone numbers is included.

Budish, Armond D. *Avoiding the Medicare Trap*. New York: Henry Holt and Co., 1989. 232p. $25.95. ISBN 0-8050-1035-1.

The author has written a sure-to-be-controversial book on how to pay for nursing-home care. An excellent chapter on who pays the bill is followed by concise, realistic advice on when Medicaid will pay for nursing-home care, and how much income an older person can keep and still qualify for Medicaid. For example, Budish presents tables showing which states have no limit on income for older individuals seeking Medicaid coverage for nursing-home costs, which have $1,062 limits, and which have limits below $1,062, as well as a state-by-state analysis of rules for protecting a person's house while he or she is in a nursing home. Additional chapters include such provocative advice as how to get around Medicaid's rules and hide assets, changing one's will and title property, and getting a divorce as a last resort for protecting assets. Budish also covers such important topics as creating living wills and finding the right lawyer.

Carper, Jean. *Health Care USA*. Englewood Cliffs, NJ: Prentice-Hall, 1987. 654p. $19.95. ISBN 0-13-609694-8.

Health Care USA is a comprehensive source book for medical and health problems. It gives names, addresses, and phone numbers from across the country for doctors, hospitals, clinics, research centers, professional and self-help centers, alternative-treatment centers, and government health agencies. Hotlines for 120 medical and health problems include information on Alz-

heimer's disease, arthritis, depression, digestive disorders, eye
and hearing problems, and heart and cardiovascular disease.

Center for Consumer Healthcare Information. *Case Management
Resource Guide,* 3 vols. Irvine, CA: Center for Consumer Healthcare
Information, 1989. 2,100p. $225 for all 3 vols., $95 per vol. ISBN
0-9624105-0-0 (3-vol. set).

> The *Resource Guide* is a first-of-its-kind, comprehensive direc-
> tory of health-care programs published in three geographic vol-
> umes (Eastern, Western, and Central South), each covering
> approximately one-third of the country. The guides cover impor-
> tant health services for consumers of all ages, including home
> care, rehabilitation services, psychiatric treatment programs, and
> addiction treatment programs. Of particular value to profession-
> als working with seniors, services needed by geriatric clients, such
> as skilled-nursing facilities and adult day care, are emphasized.
>
> The guides are impressively comprehensive, covering difficult-
> to-find services such as home modification programs and com-
> puter databases. For each entry the following information is
> provided: name and address, service area, structure (freestand-
> ing, proprietary, and date when founded, for example), parent
> organization, contact person, type of staff, how referrals are
> made, other services provided, special programs, type of quality
> assurance provided, and type of payment required. An alphabet-
> ical index to organizations and a glossary are included. The
> volumes are particularly useful for information centers, health-
> care planners, case managers, and discharge planners.

Consumer Guide. *Getting the Most from Social Security, Medicare and
Other Government Benefits.* New York: Signet, 1988. 224p. $3.50.
ISBN 0-451-15579-3.

> This *Consumer Guide* publication gives a good overview of gov-
> ernment benefit programs and related issues of importance to
> seniors. Topics include Medicare and medigap coverage. Unfor-
> tunately, important information on Medicare is outdated, but it
> is to be hoped that *Consumer Guide* is updating this affordable
> and easy-to-read book.

Crichton, Jean. *Age Care Sourcebook: A Resource Guide for the Aging
and Their Families.* New York: Simon and Schuster Inc., 1987. 335p.
$10.95. ISBN 0-671-61148-8.

The *Age Care Sourcebook* is written for elderly persons and their families to provide an easy understanding of a full range of issues to be considered regarding aging. It is easy to read, although the print is relatively small. Topics include health care, Medicare and supplemental insurance, long-term care, home health care, nursing homes, and hospice care. The book includes easy-to-use charts and an unfortunately out-of-date listing of state and area agencies on aging. Crichton's chapter covering Medicare is also outdated. A section on tips for buying supplemental health insurance is included.

Ellison, James W. *Retiring on Your Own Terms*. New York: Crown Publishers, 1989. 209p. $16.95. ISBN 0-517-57130-7.

James Ellison's retirement-planning guide covers a wide range of topics with a brief section on the hard facts of health care for retirees. The guide explains Medicare's prospective payment system and includes thoughtful information on HMOs. It is limited in other important areas: it does not include information on long-term-care insurance and provides only a brief description of Medicaid.

Health Care Education Associates. *Insurance Needs for Recipients of Medicare (INFORM): Consumer Guide* and *Insurance Needs for Recipients of Medicare (INFORM): Workshop Guide*. Laguna Niguel, CA: HealthCare Education Associates, 1989. *Consumer Guide*: 66p., $10.95. *Workshop Guide*: 160p., $79.95.

These two publications are guides to a comprehensive education program developed by HealthCare Education Associates (HCEA) to increase consumer awareness of long-term-care insurance. The project was funded by the HCFA. The *Consumer Guide* is for retirees and their families, and the *Workshop Guide* can be used by counselors, employee-benefits managers, and so on.

Inlander, Charles B., and Charles K. McKay. *Medicare Made Easy*. Reading, MA: Addison-Wesley, 1989. 336p. $10.95. ISBN 0-201-17269-0.

This excellent, accessible, comprehensive guide to Medicare is presently being updated by the authors to reflect recent changes in Medicare. The guide is a People's Medical Society Book, and the lead author is president of the society. A particularly valuable chapter covers negotiating with a doctor. An extensive appendix includes a state-by-state guide to durable power of attorney forms and living wills, valuable address lists, and a glossary.

Jehle, Faustin F. *The Complete & Easy Guide to Social Security & Medicare*. Charlotte, VT: Williamson, 1989. 172p. $9.95. ISBN 0-939945-01-7.

> The new edition of *The Complete & Easy Guide to Social Security & Medicare* is easy to read and follow. It explains Social Security, Medicare, and supplemental insurance benefits but unfortunately includes outdated information about Medicare. The guide also includes useful copies of the various forms used in applying for benefits.

Kapp, Marshall B. *Legal Aspects of Health Care for the Elderly: An Annotated Bibliography*. Westport, CT: Greenwood, 1988. 166p. $39.95. ISBN 0-313-26159-8.

> *Legal Aspects of Health Care for the Elderly* is an annotated list of 617 titles covering the period from 1980 to 1987. The author focuses on sources that cover the legal aspects of delivery of health services for the elderly. Sections of the book are valuable for coverage of such issues as elder abuse and informed consent. However, the book was written prior to passage of several important pieces of legislation that are having dramatic impact on the delivery of health services to the elderly.

Kingson, Eric. *What You Must Know about Social Security and Medicare*. New York: Pharos Books, 1987. 112p. $4.95. ISBN 0-345-34397-2.

> While Eric Kingson's highly respected simple-language guide to Social Security and Medicare is outdated, many aspects of the book remain useful to the older health consumer. It aptly describes the difference between Medicare and Medicaid and includes an excellent section on the future of Social Security and Medicare.

Matthews, Joseph L., and Dorothy M. Berman. *Social Security, Medicare and Pensions*. Berkeley, CA: Nolo Press Self-Help Law, 1990. c. 240p. $15.95. ISBN 0-87337-076-7.

Social Security, Medicare and Pensions is an easy-to-read guide to government benefit programs. Nolo Press publishes a new edition as laws change. It covers Medicare, Medicaid, Railroad Retirement, and veterans' benefits plus important information on private supplemental insurance. The guide includes illustrations and examples. The new edition describes the changes made in the Medicare law since the Medicare Catastrophic Coverage Act was repealed.

Mayer, Thomas R., and Gloria Gilbert Mayer. *The Health Insurance Alternative, A Complete Guide to Health Maintenance Organizations.* New York: Perigree, 1984. 192p. $9.95. ISBN 0-399-50979-8.

Mayer and Mayer's guide is written for a general audience, but it is useful to older health consumers because of the practical information it provides on such issues as what HMOs have to offer, their special and supplemental features, and their disadvantages. The guide has a useful table comparing the benefits a Medicare recipient would receive under a traditional fee-for-service plan and an HMO. *The Health Insurance Alternative* includes a section on special benefits for the elderly. However, information on Medicare is outdated.

Money Magazine Editors (compiled and edited by Junius Ellis). *Money 1989.* Birmingham, AL: Oxmoor House, 1989. 207p. $12.95. ISBN 0-8487-0752-4.

The emphasis of this comprehensive, beautifully designed guide is on how to build for the future. It includes sections on HMOs, choosing life-care communities, purchasing long-term-care insurance, and buying drugs by mail—all relevant to older health consumers. It also covers Medicare and medigap insurance.

Myers, Teresa Schwab. *How To Keep Control of Your Life after 60.* Lexington, MA: Lexington, 1989. 428p. $28.95. ISBN 0-669-19456-5.

Although the title does not suggest it, *How To Keep Control of Your Life after 60* focuses exclusively on legal issues affecting the elderly. Chapter Three of the book covers basic information on medigap and long-term-care insurance and a cursory chapter, "The Medicare/Medicaid Maze," provides a brief glimpse of Medicare, Medicaid, and other government benefits. Unfortunately, the information on Medicare is outdated due to repeal of the Medicare Catastrophic Coverage Act. Other chapters of interest include "Paying for Nursing Home Care," "Powers of Attorney and Other Ways of Planning Ahead," and "Guardians and Conservators: When, If and How."

National Association for Home Care (NAHC). *1990 National Homecare and Hospice Directory*. Washington, DC: NAHC, 1990. Available from NAHC. $75 for members, $200 for nonmembers.

> NAHC's directory is a detailed guide to the nation's home-care and related services. It is particularly useful for discharge planners, case managers, and other health professionals.

Neuman, R. Emil. *The Complete Handbook of U.S. Government Benefits*. Leucadia, CA: United Research, 1989. 325p. $9.95. ISBN 0-9614924-2-2.

> Emil Neuman's handbook is a guide to the full range of government benefits available to Americans of all ages. The author includes brief chapters on collecting Medicare benefits and obtaining legal help through the Legal Services Corporation.

Pearman, William A., and P. Starr. *A Handbook on the History and Issues of Health Care Services for the Elderly*. New York: Garland, 1988. 158p. $22. ISBN 0-8240-8391-1.

> This handbook is a useful reference to the history of the Medicare program. It includes a review essay, a bibliography, journal articles, government documents, unpublished papers, and an annotated bibliography of *New York Times* articles.

Pell, Arthur R., Ph.D. *Making the Most of Medicare: A Guide through the Medicare Maze*. New York: Prentice-Hall, 1987. 123p. $10.95. ISBN 0-13-547696-8.

> *Making the Most of Medicare* is an easy-to-follow guide to Medicare. It provides step-by-step assistance through several complicated and important health-consumer practices, including choosing a doctor and collecting benefits for health care. The author clearly explains Medicare, how to file claims, and how to request an appeal when a beneficiary is dissatisfied. Some of the information on Medicare is outdated. However, there is also valuable information on selecting a nursing home or home care service, choosing supplemental health insurance or a Health

Maintenance Organization, and eligibility for Medicaid or veterans' benefits. The appendix includes a listing of where to send
Medicare claims for each state and a list of medical assistance
services by state.

Regan, John J. *Your Legal Rights in Later Life*. Glenview, IL: American
Association of Retired Persons and Scott, Foresman and Co., 1989.
321p. $13.95. ISBN 0-673-24884-4.

In *Your Legal Rights in Later Life,* John J. Regan covers the legal
aspects of Medicare, Medicaid, and long-term care in a full range
of age-related topics. The guide includes question-and-answer
sections that do an excellent job of answering seniors' questions
on important legal issues. Unfortunately, some information on
Medicare is outdated.

Rubin, Leona G. *Your 1989/90 Guide to Social Security Benefits*. New
York: Facts on File, 1989. 181p. $9.95. ISBN 0-8160-2000-0.

Leona Rubin's guide includes information on Medicare that is
outdated due to repeal of the Medicare Catastrophic Coverage
Act. Much of the information is in question-and-answer format.
The author briefly covers Medicaid. The publication includes a
very useful chart comparing beneficiary expenses for Medicare
Part B under four supplemental health-insurance plans. The
chart clearly shows the value of purchasing policies that pay 40
to 100 percent of the usual and customary charge.

Schneider, Ira S., and Ezra Huber. *Financial Planning for Long-Term
Care*. New York: Human Sciences Press, 1989. 240p. $24.95. ISBN
0-89885-417-2.

Schneider and Huber's guide provides detailed information on
Medicare and Medicaid. The section on Medicaid includes useful material on third-party liability, liens and recoveries, and
transfer of assets. The authors have included in-depth information on how to appeal claims and a separate section on Medicare
that is outdated. The publication lists state Medicaid agencies.

Shane, Dorlene V. *Finances after 50: Financial Planning for the Rest of
Your Life*. New York: Harper and Row, 1989. 206p. $10.95. ISBN
0-06-096231-3.

In this practical self-study guide the author offers advice to help readers organize and manage every aspect of their financial situations including health insurance. Each section is devoted to one topic and has work sheets with easy-to-follow instructions.

Spitzer-Resnick, Jeffrey. *Your Real Medicare Handbook*. Madison, WI: Center for Public Presentation, 1987. 91p. $8. ISBN 0-932622-10-0.

In *Your Real Medicare Handbook,* Jeffrey Spitzer-Resnick offers practical information and tips on all areas of Medicare. The handbook includes valuable information on when a Medicare appeal would be most appropriate. It also includes examples of the forms that must be used when dealing with Medicare's complicated reimbursement system. Hopefully, Spitzer-Resnick is updating the *Real Medicare Handbook* to reflect recent changes in Medicare.

Thomsett, Michael. *Insurance Dictionary*. Jefferson, NC: McFarland, 1989. 243p. $29.95. ISBN 0-89950-391-8.

Michael Thomsett's easy-to-read, comprehensive dictionary of insurance terms is useful for health consumers who are not insurance-industry insiders but want to understand its jargon. The terms cover all types of insurance, and definitions usually include examples.

United Seniors Health Cooperative. *Managing Your Health Care Finances*. Washington, DC: United Seniors Health Cooperative, 1989. 71p. Price not listed. ISBN 0-994847-05-6.

The United Seniors guide to Medicare and Medicare supplements includes a guide to organizing medical bills and suggestions for an effective bill-paying system, a useful explanation of appealing Medicare claims, and tips for saving money on health-care expenses. However, its section on choosing a supplemental policy leaves out a number of important points. For example, the section doesn't mention excess charges, which can be one of the most important aspects of selecting a Medicare supplement. The guide would be highly useful if used in conjunction with the June 1989 issue of *Consumer Reports,* which is a highly recommended, comprehensive, and practical guide to choosing a Medicare supplement.

Waller, Kal. *How To Recover Your Medical Expenses*. Cleveland, OH: J. B. Zubal, 1987. 146p. $9.95. ISBN 0-939738-92-9.

> Kal Waller provides information on who is eligible for Medicare coverage and how to apply for benefits. The book gives details regarding what Medicare covers and the appeals process. However, the information on Medicare is outdated. A chapter on supplemental insurance includes checklists and work sheets to use in choosing the best supplemental coverage. A list of insurance companies by state is included, but it basically covers Blue Cross and Blue Shield insurers.

Pamphlets

> See Chapter 10, "Directory of Organizations," for addresses of the organizations whose publications are listed below.

American Association of Retired Persons Health Advocacy Services Program Department. *Before You Buy, A Guide to Long-Term Care Insurance*. 1987. 24p. Free.

> AARP's publication on long-term-care insurance describes what to look for when purchasing such care and a checklist for comparing the provisions of various policies.

———. *Choosing an HMO*. 1986. Free.

> This publication is a guide to comparing differences among HMO benefits and services and to identifying the HMOs that are adapting their system to meet the special needs of older consumers. The guide offers a step-by-step method of identifying whether an HMO is best to meet individual needs.

———. *Knowing Your Rights*. 1986. 16p. Free.

> This valuable publication provides information on Medicare's prospective payment system from a consumer point of view. It explains what the system is and describes Peer Review Organizations and appeals. A listing of the Peer Review Organizations by state is included.

American Council of Life Insurance and the Health Association of America. *Health Care and Finances: A Guide for Adult Children and Their Parents*. Not priced.

This guide is useful for its health-planning checklist for adult children to use when helping their parents plan how to pay for their health care.

Brookdale Center on Aging of Hunter College, Institute on Law and Rights of Older Adults. *Checklist for Comparing Long-Term Care Insurance—1988.* $5.

The center's checklist is useful to beneficiaries for comparing long-term-care policies.

————. (Prepared by Andrew Koski, C.S.W.) *Checklist for Purchasing Medicare Supplement Health Insurance—1989.* $1.

The center's checklist is useful to beneficiaries for comparing medigap policies.

————. *Medicare—1989.* $5.

The center's handbook on Medicare is a useful overview of the laws, regulations, benefits, and administrative appeals procedures of Medicare. The center revises the handbook yearly.

Health Care Financing Administration, Department of Health and Human Services. *Guide to Health Insurance for People with Medicare.* Free.

Discusses what Medicare pays and does not pay, describes the types of health insurance to supplement Medicare, and provides hints on shopping for insurance.

————. *Hospice Benefits under Medicare.* Free.

Describes the scope of medical and support services available to Medicare beneficiaries with terminal illness.

————. *Medicare and Employer Health Plans.* Free.

Explains the law that requires employers to offer employees age 65 and older the same health insurance they offer their younger employees.

————. *Medicare and Prepayment Plans.* Free.

Describes the services available for Medicare beneficiaries in HMO and related plans.

————. *The Medicare Handbook.* Updated annually. Free.

> The *Medicare Handbook* is a comprehensive reference guide to the Medicare program. There is an alphabetical index to assist readers. Because there are changes to the program each year, beneficiaries should request a copy annually from the closest Social Security office.

Health Insurance Association of America (HIAA). *The Consumer's Guide to Long-Term Care Insurance.* 11p. Free.

> This guide explains what long-term care is, who will need it, its expenses, and the type of insurance coverages available. A checklist for evaluating policies is included.

————. *The Consumer's Guide to Medicare Supplement Insurance.* 20p. Free.

> HIAA's guide includes a consumer's bill of rights and a checklist for consumer protection. HIAA will update the guide to reflect recent changes in Medicare.

Legal Counsel for the Elderly (LCE). *Medicare Series* (four books). 1984. $4.95 each, $15.95 set of 4.

> LCE's four guides to Medicare provide practical information in easy-to-understand language. Some of the information is outdated, however. Book One of the series covers who is eligible for Medicare, how to apply, and what to do if the beneficiary is told he or she no longer is eligible. Book Two discusses general problems such as overpayment of benefits and when benefits can be terminated. Book Three explains how to assure maximum coverage for Part A services and what to do when Medicare won't pay what it should. Book Four covers how to assure maximum coverage for doctor and outpatient services.

National Consumers League. *Medicare Handbook.* $4.

> This useful Medicare guide will be even more valuable when updated to reflect recent changes in Medicare. The handbook touches on the need for medigap insurance.

Older Women's League (OWL). *Health Insurance Continuation.* Free.

> OWL's easy-to-read publication, *Health Insurance Continuation,* provides important information about health insurance for workers and the unemployed.

Articles

Consumer Reports. *Beyond Medicare.* Reprint of article in *Consumer Reports* 54, no. 6 (June 1989): 375–391.

> This ground-breaking article provides background information on Medicare and how to choose a Medicare supplement. It succinctly explains the most important concerns of consumers shopping for Medicare supplements—coverage of excess charges and renewability. The article also provides a realistic analysis of how much a comprehensive insurance package will cost, and it rates policies sold by 25 companies representing about 80 percent of the market. It also presents an arresting exposé of insurance companies' tricks of the trade and the lack of state regulation of Medicare supplemental policies. Reprints may be obtained by writing CU/Reports, P.O. Box CS 2010-A, Mount Vernon, NY 10551.

———. *Who Can Afford a Nursing Home?* Reprint of article in *Consumer Reports* 53, no. 5 (May 1988): 300–311.

> *Who Can Afford a Nursing Home?* provides background information on the costs of long-term care and the long-term-care insurance industry. The article analyzes and compares 53 long-term-care policies. The results of the analysis can be summed up with this quote: "Many of the policies we looked at were very expensive, severely limited in their coverage, or both." The article also aptly describes the "crazy quilt of charges, waivers, and limitations that confuse even the insurance agents who try to sell the policies" and presents an excellent analysis of what long-term-care insurance policies cover and what they don't. A useful checklist of what good policies offer is also included. Reprints may be obtained by writing CU/Reports, P.O. Box CS 2010-A, Mount Vernon, NY 10551.

Periodicals

Health Letter
Public Citizen Health Research Group
2000 P Street, NW
Washington, DC 20036
Monthly, $18/year

Public Citizen's *Health Letter* covers topics relating to taking care of personal health and gaining access to "the best health care possible." Most issues include a monthly report on Medicare. Recent issues have covered the following topics relating to Medicare: catastrophic coverage, Medicare doctors denied payment for poor care, doctors dropped from Medicare, unnecessary procedures, and Medicare out-of-pocket costs.

Medicare and Medicaid Guide
Commerce Clearing House
4025 West Peterson Avenue
Chicago, IL 60646
Biweekly, about $750/year

This loose-leaf publication provides continually updated summaries of legislation, regulations, and court cases affecting Medicare and Medicaid.

United Seniors Health Report
United Seniors Health Cooperative (USHC)
Suite 500
1334 G Street, NW
Washington, DC 20005
Bimonthly, $10/year

This informative newsletter provides up-to-date information on changes in the aging network and how they affect older consumers. Recent editions have delved into the catastrophic legislation, offered advice on medigap insurance, and reported the results of a study on long-term-care insurance carried out by USHC and the University of North Carolina. The publication is a good source of information on private health-care services and developments in government legislation.

State Health Notes
Intergovernmental Health Policy Project (IHPP)
Suite 200
2011 I Street, NW
Washington, DC 20006
Contact John Sulsa for subscription information.

State Health Notes, a monthly newsletter, focuses entirely on the health-related activities of state governments. It is a particularly valuable source of information on state Medicaid programs.

State Publications on Medicare, Supplemental Plans, and Long-Term-Care Insurance

The publications listed below are free or inexpensive. They may be ordered by writing the appropriate organizations.

California

Preventing Medigap Abuse
California Department of Insurance
100 Van Ness Avenue
San Francisco, CA 94102

> *Preventing Medigap Abuse* advises older Californians on common medigap abuses and illegal methods used by some insurance agents to sell medigap insurance policies. It includes helpful forms for Medicare beneficiaries to use with their insurance agents when selecting supplemental health insurance.

Buyer's Guide to Medicare Supplemental Insurance for Californians
California Department of Insurance
100 Van Ness Avenue
San Francisco, CA 94102

> The *Buyer's Guide to Medicare Supplemental Insurance for Californians* is a comprehensive guide to Medicare's benefit gaps and supplemental health insurance. It includes a comparison of close to a hundred supplemental policies available in the state. Check with the California Department of Insurance to see whether the guide has been updated.

Long Term Care Insurance: A Consumer Guide for Californians
California Department of Insurance
100 Van Ness Avenue
San Francisco, CA 94102

> California's consumer guide to long-term-care insurance is a well-written, informative document for seniors who are considering purchasing such coverage. It includes warnings and guidelines to follow when shopping for long-term-care insurance and a valuable checklist to use in comparing policies.

Colorado

Medicare Training Manual
Senior Health Insurance Counseling Program (SHIC-P)
Colorado Gerontological Society
P.O. Box 18221
Denver, CO 80218

> SHIC-P's manual is an information resource for senior-health-insurance counselors and professionals who work with older clients or their children. Well researched and thorough, the manual is arranged in a question-and-answer format.

Connecticut

Filling in the Gaps: Health Insurance for People with Medicare
State of Connecticut
Department of Consumer Protection
165 Capital Avenue
Hartford, CT 06106

> *Filling in the Gaps* describes Medicare and its gaps with options for supplementing Medicare in Connecticut. The guide also includes sections on Medicaid; Connecticut's Prescription Aid Program, which helps eligible seniors and disabled residents by paying part of the costs of their prescriptions; the Nursing Home Preadmission Screening Program, which will coordinate and pay for home care services when a cost-effective plan of care can be offered as an alternative to institutionalization; the Center for Medicare Advocacy, which provides legal advice to elderly and disabled residents who are unfairly denied Medicare coverage; the Legal Assistance to Medicare Patients (LAMP) program, which provides attorneys to represent individuals who have been denied Medicare coverage; and the Connecticut Medicare Assignment Program (Medical Courtesy Card), which assists older adults with paying their doctor bills. Check with Connecticut's Department of Consumer Protection to see whether the publication has been updated.

Florida

Medicare Supplement Insurance Shoppers' Guide
Florida Department of Insurance
The Capital
Tallahassee, FL 32399-0300

> Florida's *Medicare Supplement Insurance Shopper's Guide* includes consumer tips on shopping for supplemental health insurance, a glossary, a guide to long-term-care insurance, and a list of companies that are licensed to sell Medicare supplemental insurance in Florida. Check with the Florida Department of Insurance to see whether it has published a new guide. The Department of Insurance also publishes a guide to health maintenance organizations.

Georgia

Georgia Nursing Home Insurance Facts
Warren D. Evans, Commissioner of Insurance
Georgia Insurance Department
716 West Tower, Floyd Building
2 Martin Luther King, Jr., Drive
Atlanta, GA 30334

> Georgia's *Nursing Home Insurance Facts* is a one-page flyer that provides a brief list of tips to follow when shopping for nursing-home insurance.

Iowa

Evaluating Nursing Home Insurance
North Central Regional Extension Publications
Publications Office, Cooperative Extension Service
Iowa State University
112 Printing and Publishing Building
Ames, IA 50011

> *Evaluating Nursing Home Insurance* is an excellent guide to evaluating personal resources and policies to cover nursing-home costs. It offers such practical advice as: "A special savings account or investment plan started before retirement could provide the

necessary funds for a nursing home stay 10, 20, or 30 years down the road. If, starting at age 55, you put $40 a month in a savings account paying 6 percent interest, you will have accumulated $28,000 by age 80. And unlike nursing home insurance, if you never require nursing home care, these funds will be available for other use."

Iowa Senior Citizens' Handbook
Iowa Department of Elder Affairs
236 Jewett Building
914 Grand Avenue
Des Moines, IA 50309

Iowa's handbook for seniors covers a broad range of issues of interest to the state's senior citizens. It includes information about Medicare, Medicaid, Medicare supplemental insurance, long-term-care facilities, elder abuse, financial materials, and other topics affecting senior citizens. Check with the Iowa Department of Elder Affairs to see whether the guide has been updated.

Kansas

Kansas Cancer Insurance Facts To Help You
Fletcher Bell, Commissioner of Insurance
State of Kansas
420 SW Ninth
Topeka, KS 66612-1678

Kansas Cancer Insurance Facts To Help You is a small brochure to assist in the purchase of cancer policies, with information on the various policies offered.

Kansas Health Insurance Facts To Help Senior Citizens
Fletcher Bell, Commissioner of Insurance
State of Kansas
420 SW Ninth
Topeka, KS 66612-1678

Kansas Health Insurance Facts To Help Senior Citizens provides basic information about Medicare and the types of health insurance available to supplement Medicare. It includes a glossary and a series of useful questions and answers addressing important health-insurance topics for seniors, such as: "Should you purchase additional policies to supplement Medicare?" and "If questions and answers arise concerning Medicare, who should you contact?" Check with the State of Kansas Insurance Commission to see whether the booklet has been updated.

Kansas Long Term Care Shopper's Guide
Fletcher Bell, Commissioner of Insurance
State of Kansas
420 SW Ninth
Topeka, KS 66612-1678

> The *Kansas Long Term Care Shopper's Guide* provides basic facts on long-term-care insurance for Kansas residents. It explains the Kansas Long Term Care Insurance Act and compares policies available for sale in Kansas, although the comparison charts are not as informative as many offered in other states.

Kansas Medicare Supplement Insurance Shopper's Guide
Fletcher Bell, Commissioner of Insurance
State of Kansas
420 SW Ninth
Topeka, KS 66612-1678

> The *Kansas Medicare Supplement Insurance Shopper's Guide* explains Medicare's basic benefits and gaps and compares the cost and coverage of Medicare-supplement policies offered by licensed companies selling approved coverage in Kansas. Check with the State of Kansas Insurance Commission to see whether the booklet has been updated.

Kentucky

Can You Afford Nursing Home Care?
Kentucky Association of Health Care Facilities
P.O. Box 692
Frankfort, KY 40602

> *Can You Afford Nursing Home Care?* is designed to inform Kentucky residents of the availability of long-term-care insurance and the limitation of this coverage under Medicare. While too

brief to be very informative, it does offer some useful tips, such as: "Annual premiums range from $200 to $2,000 and up, depending on the age at which you purchase the policy. Premium costs start to increase most dramatically when purchased after age 65. This often means insurance coverage isn't an affordable option for many elderly persons."

Maine

Consumer Long-Term Care Insurance Comparison Chart
Maine Committee on Aging
State House Station 127
Augusta, ME 04333

Maine's *Consumer Long-Term Care Insurance Comparison Chart* compares long-term-care insurance policies available in the state. However, it provides only limited guidance on how to use the chart and how to choose the best policy.

Consumer's Guide to Long-Term Care Insurance and Nursing Home Insurance in Maine
Maine Bureau of Insurance
State House Station 34
Augusta, ME 04333

This brief brochure covering long-term-care insurance provides useful information adapted from guides produced by the Health Insurance Association of America, the National Association of Insurance Commissioners, and the U.S. Department of Health and Human Services.

Medicare Supplement Insurance Comparison Chart
Maine Bureau of Insurance
State House Station 34
Augusta, ME 04333

The *Medicare Supplement Insurance Comparison Chart* explains the basics that supplemental policies must cover in the state of Maine and is a useful aid for comparing policies for sale in the state. Check with Maine's Bureau of Insurance to see whether the chart has been updated.

Maryland

Medicare & Medigap
Maryland Office on Aging
301 West Preston Street
Baltimore, MD 21201

Maryland Insurance Division
Consumer Affairs Unit
501 St. Paul Place
Baltimore, MD 21202-2272

> Maryland's consumer guide to Medicare and medigap insurance
> describes the basic components of the Medicare program and
> Maryland's minimum standards for supplemental policies. Also
> covered are useful tips on choosing policies, the rights of Medi-
> care beneficiaries, appealing claims, long-term-care insurance,
> and comparisons of supplemental policies available for sale in
> Maryland. Check with Maryland's insurance division to see
> whether the guide has been updated.

Massachusetts

Health Maintenance Organizations
Elder Affairs
Commonwealth of Massachusetts
38 Chauncy Street
Boston, MA 02111

> *Health Maintenance Organizations* outlines the advantages and
> disadvantages of HMOs as a medigap option, including a useful
> checklist of questions to ask in terms of their convenience, cost,
> and quality. The document includes comparisons of the premi-
> ums for 14 HMOs.

Long-Term Care Insurance: A Survival Guide
Elder Affairs
Commonwealth of Massachusetts
38 Chauncy Street
Boston, MA 02111

> *Long-Term Care Insurance: A Survival Guide* provides basic
> information about long-term-care insurance, including impor-
> tant questions to ask before purchasing a policy and a valuable

glossary of long-term-care insurance terms. The publication presents a thorough analysis of policies available for sale in the state, comparing such features as coverage of Alzheimer's disease and age of eligibility.

Medicare Ban on Balance Billing Law
Elder Affairs
Commonwealth of Massachusetts
38 Chauncy Street
Boston, MA 02111

> *Medicare Ban on Balance Billing Law* is a single page describing the Massachusetts law that limits the amount doctors can charge Medicare beneficiaries.

Medicare Misunderstandings
Elder Affairs
Commonwealth of Massachusetts
38 Chauncy Street
Boston, MA 02111

> *Medicare Misunderstandings* describes Medicare, its benefits, and its limitations. It also includes a useful glossary. Check with the Massachusetts Department of Elder Affairs to see whether it has been updated.

Supplementing Medicare
Elder Affairs
Commonwealth of Massachusetts
38 Chauncy Street
Boston, MA 02111

> *Supplementing Medicare* is a set of tables comparing Medicare supplemental policies for sale in Massachusetts. Check with the Massachusetts Department of Elder Affairs to see whether the tables have been updated.

Minnesota

Filling the Medicare Gaps
Minnesota Legal Services Coalition
908 Minnesota Building
St. Paul, MN 55101

> *Filling the Medicare Gaps* explains the benefits of Medicare and the options available for filling Medicare's gaps.

Mississippi

Cancer Insurance Facts To Help You
Mississippi Department of Insurance
804 Walter Sillers Building
P.O. Box 79
Jackson, MS 39205-0079

> *Cancer Insurance Facts To Help You* furnishes basic information on cancer policies and their benefits and limitations.

Health Insurance Facts To Help Senior Citizens
Mississippi Department of Insurance
1804 Walter Sillers Building
P.O. Box 79
Jackson, MS 39205-0079

> *Health Insurance Facts To Help Senior Citizens* is a brochure providing basic information on Medicare and options for supplementing it, including a brief glossary and a question-and-answer section. Check with the Mississippi Department of Insurance to see whether the publication has been updated.

Missouri

Community Leaders Assisting the Insured of Missouri (CLAIM)
State of Missouri
Division of Insurance
P.O. Box 690
Jefferson City, MO 65102-0690

> *CLAIM* is a brochure describing Missouri's network of volunteers who are trained to take insurance complaints and inquiries from consumers.

Guide to Long Term Care Insurance
Missouri Division of Insurance
P.O. Box 690
Jefferson City, MO 65102-0690

> *Guide to Long Term Care Insurance* describes the role of insurance in paying for long-term care, with factors to review and questions to ask when comparing long-term-care policies. A brief glossary is included.

Insurance Fraud Advice for Older Missourians
Special Investigative Unit
P.O. Box 690
Jefferson City, MO 65102-0690

> *Insurance Fraud Advice for Older Missourians* is a one-page brochure providing information on insurance fraud and how to identify it.

Montana

Montana Buyer's Guide to Medicare Supplement Insurance
State of Montana Insurance Commission
Sam W. Mitchell Building
P.O. Box 4009
Helena, MT 59604

> The *Montana Buyer's Guide to Medicare Supplement Insurance* provides brief definitions, tips for purchasing policies, and detailed comparisons of supplemental policies for sale to Montana Medicare beneficiaries. Check with the Montana Insurance Commission to see whether the guide has been updated.

Nebraska

Health Insurance and the Senior Citizen
Nebraska Department of Insurance
Terminal Building
941 "O" Street, Suite 400
Lincoln, NE 68508

> Medicare and the options for supplementing it are discussed in *Health Insurance and the Senior Citizen*. A checklist for use in evaluating policies is included, but it does not provide room for comparing two or more policies and is far less useful than the charts provided by a number of other states. Check with the Nebraska Department of Insurance to see whether the guide has been updated.

Long-Term Care Insurance Buyer's Guide
Nebraska Department of Insurance
Terminal Building
941 "O" Street, Suite 400
Lincoln, NE 68508

Nebraska's *Long-Term Care Insurance Buyer's Guide* includes long-term-care insurance, the conditions for coverage, points to consider when purchasing policies, and a brief glossary.

Nevada

Is Medicare Enough?—A Shoppers' Guide to Supplemental Medical Insurance
Commissioner of Insurance
State of Nevada
201 South Fall Street
Carson City, NV 89710

> *Is Medicare Enough?* features a checklist for comparing insurance policies and hints to assist individuals in purchasing Medicare-supplement policies.

New Hampshire

Guide to Nursing Home (Long-Term Care) Insurance
State of New Hampshire Insurance Department
169 Manchester Street
Concord, NH 03301

> New Hampshire's *Guide to Nursing Home (Long-Term Care) Insurance* is a small brochure describing the role insurance plays in paying for long-term care, with questions to ask when shopping for policies and a brief glossary. Unfortunately, most of the information is incomplete and confusing to the reader. For example, the brochure suggests that the reader ask the following question when comparing policies: "What is the pre-existing condition limitation of this policy?" But the brochure does not define the condition limitation or explain why it is important.

New Jersey

Bridging the Medicare Gaps
Department of Insurance
201 East State Street
Trenton, NJ 08625

> New Jersey's *Bridging the Medicare Gaps* is the most comprehensive, readable, and accessible of the state publications on

Medicare and supplemental health insurance. The booklet describes Medicare and options for filling its gaps. Beautifully executed comparison charts of Medicare supplements and long-term-care policies are included. Color coding of the Medicare supplement chart makes it easy to analyze. Check with the New Jersey Department of Insurance to see whether the booklet has been updated.

New York

Medicare Supplement Insurance in New York State
State of New York Insurance Department
Agency Building One
Empire State Plaza
Albany, NY 12257

> *Medicare Supplement Insurance in New York State* is a substantial publication describing Medicare and supplements sold in the state, with detailed comparisons of policies and addresses and telephone numbers of insurers. Check with the State of New York Insurance Department to see whether the publication has been updated.

North Dakota

Nursing Home Insurance Shoppers Guide
North Dakota Insurance Department
State Capitol, Fifth Floor
Bismarck, ND 58505-0158

> North Dakota's guide to nursing-home insurance is a brief pamphlet explaining long-term care and insurance options for paying for it. It also has shopping tips, hints to follow after the consumer has chosen a policy, and a glossary.

What Insurance Policies Do Most Senior Citizens Need?
North Dakota Insurance Department
State Capitol, Fifth Floor
Bismarck, ND 58505-0158

> *What Insurance Policies Do Most Senior Citizens Need?* is a brief, cryptic document comprising a list of dos and don'ts to

take into consideration when shopping for insurance to supplement Medicare, tables delineating the Medicare program, checklists for supplemental and long-term-care insurance, and a brief glossary. Check with the North Dakota Insurance Department to see whether the publication has been updated.

Ohio

Ohio Buyer's Guide to Medicare Supplemental Health Insurance and Benefits Comparison Booklet
Ohio Department of Insurance
2100 Stella Court
Columbus, OH 43266-0566

> Ohio's guide to medigap insurance is a one-page piece explaining Medicare's gaps and providing incomplete advice on what to look for when purchasing supplemental insurance. It is more useful when used with Ohio's *Benefits Comparison Booklet*. Contact the Ohio Department of Insurance to see whether the publications have been updated.

Oregon

A Guide to Long-Term Care Insurance in the State of Oregon
Department on Insurance and Finance
21 Labor and Industries Building
Salem, OR 97310

> Oregon's guide to long-term-care insurance includes a glossary and an exhaustive collection of summaries of the long-term-care policies available for sale in the state. The summaries are updated as new policies are approved, but there is no guidance on how to use the extensive summaries. The document should be used in conjunction with a health-insurance counselor.

Pennsylvania

Comparison of Long-Term Care Insurers
Commonwealth of Pennsylvania
Department of Aging
Harrisburg, PA 17101

Pennsylvania's *Comparison of Long-Term Care Insurance* is a list of the policies available for sale in the state, including such factors as length of coverage and maximum daily benefits. However, such important information as whether a policy covers Alzheimer's disease and what its terms of renewability are is not included.

Your Guide to Long-Term Care Insurance
Commonwealth of Pennsylvania
Department of Aging
Harrisburg, PA 17101

Pennsylvania's guide to long-term-care insurance is a small brochure providing limited information for consumers shopping for such insurance. A checklist included in the back portion of the brochure is not titled, and it is unclear what use it has for the reader. Assuming it is a checklist for evaluating policies, it does have a couple of questions that are excellent, however. First, it asks the reader to gather information about the costs of nursing homes and home health care in the area and then to compare figures on how much a policy would pay and the policy's cost over time.

Rhode Island

Rhode Island Guide to Buying Medicare Supplement Insurance
Rhode Island Department of Elderly Affairs
Information and Referral Service
79 Washington Street
Providence, RI 02903-1893

Rhode Island's medigap guide, in question-and-answer format, offers information on the benefits of Medicare and tips on purchasing Medicare supplemental insurance. The document includes a comparison of supplements sold in the state and a list of the insurers selling long-term-care insurance. Check with the Rhode Island Department of Elderly Affairs to see whether the guide has been updated.

South Carolina

South Carolina Health Insurance Buyer's Guide
South Carolina Department of Insurance
2711 Middleburg Drive
Columbia, SC 29204

> Health-insurance information for consumers of all ages is provided in South Carolina's health-insurance guide, including limited information on the special needs of senior citizens.

Tennessee

Medicare, Medicaid, and Medicare Supplement Insurance: What You Need To Know To Protect Yourself
Legal Services of Middle Tennessee, Inc.
211 Union Street, Suite 800
Nashville, TN 37201

Knoxville Legal Aid Society, Inc.
502 Gay Street, Suite 404
Knoxville, TN 37902

> Tennessee is one of the few states that has included important information on Medicaid and how it works in a health insurance guide for seniors. This helpful brochure on Medicare and related topics also includes information on Medicare supplemental insurance, describing specific policies and benefits. One important section, "Policies with the Big Five Features," is introduced so far into the guide that many readers may miss it. The booklet contains valuable information on Medicare appeals. Check with Legal Services of Middle Tennessee to see whether the guide has been updated.

Texas

Medicare Supplement Insurance: A Guide for Texas Consumers
Information Services
State Board of Insurance
1110 San Jacinto Boulevard
Austin, TX 78701-1998

Medicare Supplement Insurance: A Guide for Texas Consumers provides basic information on Medicare and Medicare supplemental insurance, including the rights of seniors under Texas law. Shopping tips and sources of additional information are given, as well as a checklist for comparison shopping. Check with the State Board of Insurance to see whether the guide has been updated.

A Shopper's Guide to Long Term Care Insurance in Texas
Information Services
State Board of Insurance
1110 San Jacinto Boulevard
Austin, TX 78701-1998

The Texas guide to long-term-care insurance is a question-and-answer booklet that includes shopping tips, a glossary, and help in filing complaints. The guide has comparisons of policies and their costs, providing valuable information on such issues as coverage of Alzheimer's disease and availability of inflation protection.

Utah

A Practical Guide for Medigap Policies Offered in Utah
Utah Department of Insurance
P.O. Box 45803
Salt Lake City, UT 84145

A Practical Guide for Medigap Policies Offered in Utah is a comprehensive booklet covering valuable information about medigap policies and Medicaid plus limited information on long-term-care insurance. Included is a comparison chart of costs and benefits of the policies for sale in Utah with an excellent introduction explaining how to use it. Check with the Utah Department of Insurance to see whether the guide has been updated.

Vermont

A Consumer's Guide to Long Term Care Insurance in Vermont
Vermont Office on Aging
Agency of Human Services
State of Vermont
109 State Street
Montpelier, VT 05602

> Vermont's guide on long-term-care insurance presents a brief but valuable analysis of four major ways to pay for long-term care. Also included is a review of such insurance and a checklist for comparing policies. A comparison chart of policies sold in the state is available from the Vermont Department of Banking and Insurance.

Washington

Health Insurance Guide for Senior Citizens
Dick Marquardt, Insurance Commissioner
Insurance Building
Olympia, WA 98504

> Washington's *Health Insurance Guide for Senior Citizens* is an excellent small booklet covering important consumer information for seniors shopping for health insurance, including limited information about long-term-care insurance.

West Virginia

West Virginia Supplement Shopper's Guide
West Virginia Insurance Commissioner
2100 Washington Street, East
Charleston, WV 25305

> West Virginia's shopper's guide is an extensive set of charts comparing companies that offer supplemental health insurance in the state. It should be used with a health-insurance counselor who can provide information about the benefit options covered in the brochure.

Wisconsin

Buyer's Guide to Long Term Care
Office of the Commissioner of Insurance
P.O. Box 7873
Madison, WI 53707-7873

> Wisconsin's guide to long-term care provides only limited facts about nursing-home insurance. A list of policies available in Wisconsin may be obtained by enclosing a stamped, self-addressed envelope to the Office of the Commissioner of Insurance. The list is not as useful as many of the comparison charts offered by other states.

Health Insurance Advice for Senior Citizens
Office of the Commissioner of Insurance
P.O. Box 7873
Madison, WI 53707-7873

> The Medicare program, supplemental health insurance, and HMOs are described briefly in Wisconsin's *Health Insurance Advice for Senior Citizens*. Comparisons of individual policies sold in Wisconsin may be obtained by enclosing a stamped, self-addressed envelope to the Office of the Commissioner of Insurance. The comparison charts include a fascinating list of the amount that insurance agents make on the first year's commission on policies. For example, a number of policies give agents 50.5 percent of the premium (which may range from $500 to more than $1,000) during the first year after a policy is sold, and some are as high as 60 percent. However, Blue Cross/Blue Shield United of Wisconsin pays agents $3 as the first year's commission. Which policies do you think agents push?

Nonprint Materials

Software

Benefits Outreach Screening Software (BOSS)
Type: Menu-driven
System: IBM compatible

Source: United Seniors Health Cooperative (USHC)
            1334 G Street, NW, Suite 500
            Washington, DC 20005
            (202) 393-6222
Cost: Contact USHC

BOSS screens users for eligibility for benefit programs and produces a personalized *Benefit Check-Up* report listing programs to which the person is entitled.

Medigap Counseling Software

Type: Menu-driven
System: IBM compatible
Source: United Seniors Health Cooperative (USHC)
            1334 G Street, NW, Suite 500
            Washington, DC 20005
            (202) 393-6222
Cost: Contact USHC

This software allows an organization to compile information on the most common medigap policies purchased by older people in the community. The *Medigap Check-Up* report answers questions regarding Medicare coverage and gaps, policy features, and policy selection.

Glossary

activities of daily living (ADLs) The major daily activities of bathing, dressing, eating, and toileting. Such activities are often used to measure degree of disability.

actual charge   The amount billed by the physician or supplier for medical services or supplies. It often differs from the Medicare allowable charge.

acute disease   A disease or condition characterized by a single episode of short duration. The patient usually returns to a normal or previous state and level of activity.

administrative hearing   The second step in the Medicare appeals process, in which an administrative law judge examines evidence and takes testimony on a case.

administrative law judge   The judge who examines evidence and takes testimony in the second stage of the Medicare appeals process.

adult day care   A community service that usually provides lunch, general nursing service, and personal hygiene to impaired individuals who are being cared for by family members at home. Other services may include dietary counseling; special diets; physical, occupational, and speech therapy; psychiatric services; and transportation. The purpose of adult day care is to allow individuals to remain at home and in the community and also to encourage families to care for them by providing relief from the burden of constant care.

age at entry   The age of an insured person at the time of application or the effective date of an insurance policy.

allowed charge   Also called approved charge. *See* reasonable charge.

ambulatory centers   Health centers that provide services on an outpatient basis. The center may be affiliated with a hospital or be independent.

ancillary services   Services provided in the hospital other than room and board, such as X ray, drug, laboratory, or other variables.

appeal   The right of the physician and/or a beneficiary to question denial of payments or allowed amounts of paid benefits.

assessment   Identifying the level of impairment of an individual and the type and extent of services needed. An assessment may measure everything from social resources to health-related information.

assignment   An agreement with Medicare through which a physician or supplier will accept Medicare payment as payment in full except for the coinsurance and deductible amount. Beneficiaries do not have to pay the physician's or supplier's actual charge. Payment by Medicare is made directly to the physician or supplier.

balance billing   The difference between the total amount of the bill that is charged by the physician (or other medical provider) and the "Medicare-approved amount." Some supplemental-insurance companies will pay the excess charges and some will pay only the remaining 20 percent of the Medicare-approved amount.

basic premium amount   The base amount that Medicare uses to determine the premium for beneficiaries purchasing Medicare coverage.

Baucus Amendment   Passed in 1980 to set new standards for Medicare supplemental policies. No policy may be sold as a Medicare supplement unless it meets these standards.

beneficiary   A person who is eligible to receive or is receiving benefits from an insurance policy.

benefit maximum   The upper-limit amount an insurance policy will pay for a particular service, indicated either by a dollar amount or a period of time.

benefit period   For Medicare Part A, a benefit period begins on the day of admission to a hospital or skilled-nursing home and ends 60 days after discharge from the institution.

benefits   The services Medicare or an insurance policy will cover and what it will pay.

Best book rating   A. M. Best rates the financial stability of insurance companies. An A+ is the highest rating a company can attain.

Blue Cross   An independent corporation providing benefits, on a service basis, against the cost of hospital care in a limited geographic area.

Blue Shield   An independent corporation providing benefits, on a service basis, against the cost of medical and surgical care in a limited geographic area.

capitation   Payment method by which a health-care provider (usually a doctor) is paid a fixed amount for each person served, without regard to the kind or quantity of services provided.

carrier   A private organization that contracts with the federal government to process and pay claims covered by Medicare medical insurance (Medicare Part B).

catastrophic health insurance   Health-insurance coverage to help pay the high cost of severe or lengthy medical care.

chronic condition   A condition requiring continuation of care on an ongoing basis. Usually nonreversible in nature, it may require therapy or training for rehabilitation.

churning   The inappropriate replacement of an existing insurance policy with a new one.

claim   A request made by the insured to the insurer for payment of benefits. A claim can be filed by the insured or by the provider. In a health maintenance organization (HMO), claim forms are necessary only in the case of outside care.

claims review   The procedure by which medical care received by an insuree is checked over by the insurer to make certain that it was medically acceptable and therefore valid for payment. There is no claims-review procedure in an HMO, although other types of reviews are mandated by law. Medicare claims are handled by intermediaries or carriers under contracts with the Health Care Financing Administration (HCFA).

Competitive Medical Plans (CMPs)   Medicare calls some HMOs Competitive Medical Plans (CMPs). CMP refers to plans with a particular kind of government contract called a risk contract.

comprehensive outpatient rehabilitation facility (CORF)   Facilities providing a broad range of medical services designed for rehabilitation. Medicare has limited coverage for CORF services.

conditionally renewable   A policy phrase meaning that the company will continue to insure the beneficiary as long as it continues to insure people in the same state with the same kind of coverage.

conservator   In most states, a guardian of a ward.

coordination of benefits (COB)   A provision used by an insurance company to avoid duplication of paid benefits, particularly when a person has insurance with more than one company. Insurance companies have varying standards for determining who is the primary payer.

copayment or coinsurance   Plan in which the participant pays a portion of the recognized medical expenses. A policy that uses copayment or coinsurance typically pays up to 80 percent of a given expense and the policyholder pays the remainder (as is the case with Medicare).

cost sharing   A term used to describe Medicare provisions such as deductibles and coinsurance that require the beneficiary or policyholder to pay a certain amount of the expenses covered by Medicare.

custodial care   Services that give assistance with personal needs such as bathing, walking, and dressing and are provided by persons without professional skills or training.

deductible   An amount of expense beneficiaries must incur before insurance begins to pay benefits for covered services. The deductible must be satisfied every calendar year, although many plans have three-month carryover provisions in which the last three months of the previous year can be applied toward satisfaction of the following year's deductible.

demand billing   Also referred to as no-payment billing. The beneficiary "demands" that a Part A facility submit a claim to Medicare even though it expects no payment.

diagnosis-related grouping (DRG)   A method of payment used by Medicare to reimburse hospitals based on diagnosis rather than on hospital costs. There are 477 diagnosis-related groups (DRGs) that determine the reimbursement hospitals receive under the Prospective Payment system.

disability   A physical or mental handicap, particularly one that limits the ability to perform certain tasks.

durable medical equipment (DME)   Equipment that can stand repeated use and is utilized in the direct treatment of an illness or injury. Generally it is not helpful in the absence of illness or injury. DME includes oxygen equipment, wheelchairs, home dialysis systems, and other medically necessary equipment.

elimination period   Applies to a specific type of policy called a "hospital income policy" or "hospital indemnity policy." Benefits are not paid under the elimination period for the first several days of hospitalization. Elimination periods vary from policy to policy and company to company. The longer the elimination period, the lower the cost of the insurance, but consumers are less likely to receive benefits for a short period of illness.

entrance age   The age up to which a company will sell an individual a policy.

excess charges   Also referred to as balance billing. The difference between the total amount of the bill that is charged by the physician (or other medical provider) and the Medicare-approved amount. Some supplemental-insurance companies will pay part or all of the excess charges and some will pay only the remaining 20 percent of the Medicare-approved amount.

exclusion   A condition resulting in an illness for which the policy will not pay benefits.

federal qualification   Accreditation for HMOs that meet the requirements of the federal government's HMO laws, including stipulation of services, community rating, a board of directors that includes HMO members, health education, social services, fiscal viability, security of members, and open enrollment. Some HMOs provide these services even though they are not federally qualified, because the paperwork involved in qualification can be prohibitive.

fee-for-service   A payment system by which doctors or hospitals are paid a specific amount for each service performed. Traditional insurance benefits are paid on this basis.

first-dollar coverage   A policy that, like an HMO, has no deductibles and covers the first dollar of an insuree's expenses.

fraud   Intentional misrepresentation by either a provider of medical care or a claimant to obtain services or payment of services, or to claim eligibility. Fraud carries penalties when discovered.

free-look period   The period of time for the health-insurance consumer to look at a new policy and determine whether it is the best coverage for him or her.

generic drug   A copy of a brand-name drug manufactured by a company other than the originating company.

group HMO   An HMO that contracts with one or more independent group practices to provide services in one or more locations, in which physicians are prepaid on a capitation basis.

group insurance   An insurance plan for a number of employees or members of an organization (and their dependents) insured under a single policy. Each insured individual receives an individual certificate.

guaranteed renewable   Agreement by an insurance company to continue insuring the beneficiary up to a certain age or for life as long as he or she pays the premium. The company cannot raise premiums unless it raises them for a particular class, such as all those in a geographic area with the same kind of policy. This is the most desirable type of renewability.

guardian   The legal custodian of a ward.

health maintenance organization (HMO)   A public or private organization that provides a comprehensive range of health-care services to enrolled members. Members must live within a specified geographic area and use only specified physicians. A fee is charged that is frequently less than the cost of supplemental health insurance. There is no paperwork to file to receive services.

health screening   Requirement by a health-insurance company that an applicant complete a series of medical questions prior to approval of the policy; a medical examination by a licensed physician also may be required.

hearing   The second step in the Medicare appeal process for both Part A and Part B, in which the beneficiary may appear before a hearing officer to state his or her reasons for disagreeing with Medicare's decision on a claim. The dispute must involve more than $1,000.

homebound   A condition whereby leaving home would be medically inadvisable, could be harmful, and would involve considerable effort. Homebound is sometimes narrowly and rigidly defined as unable to leave home under any circumstances (i.e., bedbound).

home health agency   An organization that provides part-time skilled-nursing services and therapy services such as physical therapy in a patient's home.

home health care   Care provided in the person's home by a registered nurse, physical therapist, or speech therapist under the supervision of a physician.

homemaker services   Nonmedical support services (such as preparing meals and helping in bathing) provided for homebound persons.

hospice   A program that engages primarily in providing pain relief, symptom management, and supportive services for terminally ill people and their families.

hospital insurance   The portion of Medicare or health insurance that covers inpatient hospital stays, some inpatient care in a skilled-nursing facility, and home health agencies.

incapacity   Lack of the legal power to act in specified ways.

indemnity policy   A policy that pays a fixed amount for a covered service no matter what the actual cost of the service. Indemnity policies are not good options for supplementing Medicare.

informal care giving   Care giving provided by nonprofessionals such as family and friends.

inpatient care   Care provided to patients who are admitted to the hospital or nursing home for more than a day.

Insurance Commission   A division of each state's Department of Regulatory Agencies that regulates all insurance companies in each state. Commissions are responsible for licensing insurance companies and insurance agents and for collecting premium taxes and licensing fees. They also act as liaisons between consumers and the insurance industry and handle arbitration of consumer complaints regarding insurance companies.

intermediary   A private organization that contracts with the federal government to process and pay claims from hospitals, skilled-nursing facilities, home health agencies, and providers of hospice care.

intermediate nursing care   Care that is less intensive than skilled care. Generally some nursing assistance is provided around the clock. Medical treatment must be available but on an occasional basis.

intermittent   Used in relation to medical services to determine whether a patient requires skilled or intermediate services and whether a patient is eligible for Medicare home health benefits. Intermittent services are in the intermediate category.

lifetime maximum benefits   The total benefits, in time or maximum dollar amounts, that an insurance policy will ever pay.

limitation   A situation or circumstance under which an insurance policy will not pay. Limitations are usually listed with exclusions in an insurance policy.

limits on out-of-pocket expenditures   Because meeting the coinsurance and deductible amounts can pose a hardship, most insurance plans contain a limit on out-of-pocket expenditures. Once a subscriber has reached the maximum, say $5,000, covered expenses are reimbursed in full for the remainder of the year. The limit is usually renewed at the start of the calendar year for each individual participant.

long-term care   The wide range of medical and support services provided to persons who have lost some or all capacity to function on their own.

long-term-care insurance   An insurance policy to help pay for a chronic illness or disability that lasts a long time when the individual is no longer able to care for himself or herself. The services covered can include nursing-home care and home health care services. (Policies that include home health care are preferable.) Some of the better policies also cover adult day care, plus respite care (which provides time off for family members caring for an ill or disabled person at home).

loss ratio   The percentage of premiums paid out in claims. Medicare supplemental policies are required to have minimum loss ratios of 60 percent on individual policies and 75 percent on group coverage.

major medical insurance   Insurance that covers only catastrophic illness or accidents that incur large and long-term expenses.

mammography   X ray of the breast for early detection of cancer.

Medicaid (Title XIX)   A program that pays for medical benefits for low-income individuals. Medicaid is funded jointly by federal and state governments and operated and administered by the states.

medical insurance   The noninstitutional portion of Medicare or health insurance that covers physician services, outpatient hospital services, some home health services, and a number of other services and supplies.

medically necessary   Care that is appropriate, reasonable, and necessary for diagnosis or treatment as generally accepted by the professional health community. It is usually determined by the patient's physician and/or insurer or, in the case of Medicare, a Peer Review Organization and/or a Utilization Review Committee. Medicare will not pay for services that are not medically necessary.

medically needy or medically indigent   A person who is unable to pay his or her medical bills. "Medically indigent" can refer to those of low income who cannot pay for medical care or to those of adequate income who are faced with catastrophic health-care costs.

Medicare (Title XVIII)   A nationwide health-insurance program for people 65 and older, for those who have been eligible for Social Security for more than two years and are disabled, and for those suffering from end-stage renal disease.

Medicare Part A   The portion of Medicare that pays for inpatient hospital stays, skilled-nursing facilities, home health services, and hospice care.

Medicare Part B The portion of Medicare that pays for services by physicians and noninstitutional suppliers.

Medicare HMO An HMO that is certified by the HCFA to enroll Medicare beneficiaries.

Medicare-certified Health-care providers that have received approval from Medicare to provide services to beneficiaries.

medigap or supplemental insurance Private health insurance that helps to pay for hospital and medical services and supplies not paid for in full by Medicare.

network HMO An HMO that contracts with one or more independent group practices to provide services in one or more locations, in which physicians are prepaid on a capitation basis.

nonparticipating facility Facility that does not participate in the Medicare program and generally does not receive Medicare payment for services.

nonreplacement fee A fee charged by a provider of medical care for blood that is not replaced.

notice of noncoverage Written notices hospitals must give to Medicare beneficiaries when they are going to discharge them.

nurse practitioner Performs physical examinations and diagnostic tests, counsels patients, and develops treatment programs. Regulations regarding their duties vary from state to state. Nurse practitioners may work independently, such as in rural clinics, or may be staff members at hospitals and other health facilities. Medicare will help pay for services performed under the supervision of a doctor.

nursing facilities (NFs) Facilities providing around-the-clock supervision and treatment by a registered nurse under the direction of a doctor. NFs serve people who require continual medical services.

nursing home   A facility that cares for people with mental or physical limitations. Only a specific type of nursing home, a skilled-nursing home, is Medicare certified.

nursing-home ombudsman   The person responsible on a state level to receive, investigate, and act on complaints by older persons who are residents of long-term-care facilities. All states have designated ombudsmen who work through state and area agencies on aging.

Older Americans Act (OAA)   Act passed in 1965 to provide for a variety of social services and meal programs for older persons. Services are supplied through more than 600 state and area agencies on aging.

open enrollment   A period of time when an individual or member of a group may purchase insurance. For example, open enrollment for purchasing Medicare insurance is between January 1 and March 31 each year.

option   Additional coverage(s) or benefit(s) that may be added at extra cost to an insurance policy.

outliers   Under the Prospective Payment System, cases that are classified into a specific DRG but have an unusually long period of stay or high cost. Outliers allow hospitals to receive supplemental payments in addition to the normal reimbursement.

outpatient hospital service   Diagnostic and treatment health services given on an outpatient basis by a Medicare-participating hospital.

paralegal   A professional who can perform many of the tasks of a lawyer, such as public-benefits work. Paralegals are not recognized by bar associations.

participating physician   A physician who has agreed to accept assignment on all Medicare claims.

participating supplier   A supplier who has signed an agreement to accept assignment on all Medicare claims.

patient representative Hospital employee whose job it is to notify patients of their rights and help them with discharge plans.

Peer Review Organization (PRO) A group of local physicians and other professionals who are under contract with the HCFA to review the services provided by hospitals and skilled-nursing facilities, to make sure that the services meet professional standards and are as economical as possible.

period of confinement Provision in long-term-care insurance policies stipulating how long the insured person can stay out of the nursing home before having to go through a new waiting period.

physical therapy Services furnished by specially trained and licensed physical therapists to relieve pain, restore maximum function, and prevent disability, injury, or loss of a body part.

physician services Health-care services provided by a physician (or a physician's assistant under the supervision of a physician). The service may be performed in the doctor's office, a home, or a health-care facility such as a skilled-nursing home.

preadmission screening Under Medicaid a comprehensive assessment of health and social-service needs of individuals requesting Medicaid nursing-home placement, to determine whether in-home or community-based care options are feasible or desirable.

preexisting condition A current health problem that the health-insurance consumer had prior to purchasing health insurance. Most insurance companies define a preexisting condition as one that occurred within six months before the policy takes effect, but some go back as far as five years.

preferred provider organization (PPO) A group of providers that agrees to supply health-care services to holders of specific health-insurance policies or medical coverage (through an employer, insurance company, or similar group) for prenegotiated fees, usually at a reduced cost to the insurance company or organization offering the coverage.

premium   An amount of money paid for an insurance policy. Usually paid monthly, quarterly, semiannually, or annually.

prevailing charge   The maximum charge Medicare can pay for any item or service, based upon the provider's usual charge for covered medical services or items.

pro bono   From the Latin *pro bono publico,* "for the public good." The term usually means that a lawyer or firm will take a case free of charge.

Professional Standards Review Organization (PSRO)   An organization that was responsible for review of health-care services, funded by Medicare to determine whether those services are reasonable, medically necessary, furnished in an appropriate setting, and of a quality that meets professionally recognized standards. The PSRO has been replaced by Peer Review Organizations (PROs).

prospective payment system (PPS)   The system under which hospitals pay fixed amounts based on principal diagnosis for each hospital stay rather than costs. Introduced on October 1, 1983, it classifies conditions into one of 477 diagnosis-related groups (DRGs).

prosthetic devices   Devices affixed to or implanted in the body that are designed to take the place, or perform the function, of a missing body part, such as an artificial arm or leg.

provider   An individual or institution that gives medical care. In Medicare this can be an individual physician, hospital, skilled-nursing facility, home health agency, therapist, supplier of durable medical equipment, pharmacist, or other person or entity that provides medical care.

reasonable and necessary care   The amount and type of health services considered by Medicare as being necessary to treat a specific disease or illness.

reasonable charge   Also called approved or allowable charge, the amount approved by Medicare based on charges submitted to Medicare over a period of time by medical providers. It is a comparison of the *customary charge,* the *prevailing charge,* and the *current actual charge.* Payment is based on the lowest of the three.

reconsideration   The first step in the Medicare appeals process, in which the beneficiary sends a written request to the intermediary showing his or her disagreement with the decision made on a claim.

reinstated benefits   The lifetime maximum restored by some policies according to a specified schedule during periods when the beneficiary is not drawing benefits.

renewable at company option   The right reserved by a company to stop insuring clients on an individual basis. However, the company cannot terminate the policy in the midst of an illness.

replacement   Purchase of a policy by a consumer to replace one that he or she already owns.

reserve days   Medicare's lifetime allotment to every beneficiary of 60 days of hospital coverage that can be used when extended hospital care is required beyond a benefit period. The beneficiary must pay daily coinsurance.

respite care   Temporary relief for family members who are responsible for caring for an ill or disabled person at home.

rider   An attachment to an insurance policy that modifies or adds to the benefits in some way.

risk contracts   Medicare HMO contracts, one of whose features is a lock-in specifying that neither Medicare nor the HMO will pay anything if the HMO Medicare member goes to a doctor or other provider outside the HMO.

routine care   Care provided by physicians to prevent acute conditions from arising. These include such services as annual physical examinations, immunizations, and eye examinations. Medicare does not pay for routine care, and some insurance companies also do not.

second opinion   Diagnosis by a second physician confirming or differing from the findings of the first physician.

secondary payer   Medicare as payer after other insurance company's payment has been made.

skilled-nursing care   Care performed by or under the supervision of a licensed nurse or therapist and provided under the supervision of a physician. Without skilled-nursing care the individual's health would be seriously threatened.

skilled-nursing facility   A Medicare-certified facility with the staff and equipment to provide skilled-nursing care and related rehabilitative services.

Social Security Appeals Council review   The third stage in the Medicare appeals process, in which the Appeals Council in Arlington, Virginia, decides whether to hear a case, dismiss it, or send it back to an administrative law judge for review.

social services   Counseling and guidance services offering advice in emotional, psychological, financial, or legal matters and assistance in obtaining community services.

speech therapy   The study, examination, and treatment of defects and diseases of the voice, speech, and spoken and written language.

staff-based HMO   An HMO in which services are delivered at one or more locations by doctors who are employed by the HMO.

subscriber   An individual or family in whose name a health-care policy is issued.

Supplemental Security Income (SSI)   Monthly payments to people who are aged, disabled, or blind and have low incomes. Federal funds come from general revenues, not Social Security taxes. Any Social Security office can provide additional information.

supplier   An entity from which health-care consumers can purchase items such as durable medical equipment or prescription drugs.

Medicare requires suppliers to meet all licensing requirements of state and local health authorities. Suppliers must be certified by Medicare in order to be considered for payment of Medicare benefits.

surgicenter   A facility that serves outpatients requiring surgical treatment beyond what can be provided in a physician's office but not requiring an inpatient hospital stay.

swing bed   A bed in a hospital that can be used either as a hospital or skilled-nursing bed.

third-party payment   Payment for health-care services by someone other than the individual who received the care or administered it.

underwriting   In insurance, a process of setting premium rates through a procedure of selecting, classifying, evaluating, and assuming risks according to insurability. The underwriting process must classify risks into categories with about the same expectation of loss.

utilization review committee   Committee of physicians or other medical professionals in a health facility that evaluates the necessity, appropriateness, and efficiency of the use of medical services, procedures, and facilities.

vendor   An institution, agency, organization, or practitioner who provides medical services.

waiting period   A specified period of time during which a subscriber to a new policy will not be paid for a preexisting condition.

waiver of liability   Under Medicare law, a provision that a beneficiary cannot be held responsible for paying for care not covered by Medicare.

waiver of premium   A feature in some insurance policies providing that after a period when certain benefits were payable, future premium payments will be waived as long as those benefits continue to be payable. When the benefits cease, the obligation to pay subsequent premium payments resumes.

ward   An individual legally placed under the guardianship of a person or agency.

Index

A. M. Best rating for insurance, 94

AAA (Area Agencies on Aging), 115, 117, 207

AACC (American Association for Continuity of Care), 213

AAHA (American Association of Homes for the Aging), 194–198

AARP. *See* American Association of Retired Persons

Accident-only policies, 109

Administrative Hearing for Part A Medicare appeals, 65, 68

Administrative law judges, 65, 78

ADRDA (Alzheimer's Disease and Related Disorders Association), 127, 217

Adult day care, 124, 213

Adult Day Care Quarterly, 213

Adult foster care, 123

Adult protective services, 123–124

Age Care Sourcebook: A Resource Guide for the Aging and Their Families, 229–230

Agencies, government, 171–193

Aging Network Services (ANS), 117, 213

Aging Notes, 193

Agreement To Have Representative at Hearing, 80–81

AHCA (American Health Care Association), 198–201

Almond, Sherry, 227

Altman, Maya, 227

Alzheimer's Association (Alzheimer's Disease and Related Disorders Association), 127, 217

AMA (American Medical Association), 6–7

Ambulances, Medicare coverage of, 40

Ambulatory emergency centers, 143–144

Ambulatory surgical services, 39

American Association for Continuity of Care (AACC), 213

American Association of Homes for the Aging (AAHA), 194–198

American Association of Retired Persons (AARP), 161
book by, 227
home health care lawsuit by, 31
legal assistance from, 126
on long-term care, 8
MMAP program by, 16–17, 161
pamphlets by, 236

American Bar Association, 126

American Bar Association Commission on Legal Problems of the Elderly, 162

American Council of Life Insurance and the Health Association of America, 236

American Health Care Association (AHCA), 198–201

American Legion, 108

American Medical Association (AMA), 6–7

American Public Welfare Association (APWA), 214

ANS (Aging Network Services), 117, 213

Appeals, Medicare, 63–64
Part A, 65–75, 78–83
Part B, 75–83

Appeals Council Review for Part A Medicare claims, 66, 69

Application for Enrollment in Medicare, 46–48

Application To Purchase Medicare Coverage, 11–15

Approved amount for Part B Medicare services, 45

APWA (American Public Welfare Association), 214

Area Agencies on Aging (AAA), 115, 117, 207

Assets and Medicaid, 131–133

Assignment method for Part B Medicare, 46, 49–51, 102, 145
Assisted-living centers, 133
Audiologists, 158–159
Automatic retrospective reviews, 74
Avoiding the Medicare Trap, 228

Balance billing, 49, 248
Basic home health services, 118–119
Baucus Amendment, 89–90, 96
Before You Buy, A Guide to Long-Term Care Insurance, 236
Bell, Fletcher, 244–245
Bellevue Hospital, 20
Benefit maximums with supplemental insurance, 93
Benefit periods for inpatient hospital services, 23
Benefits Outreach Screening Software (BOSS), 258–259
Berko, Robert L., 227
Berman, Dorothy M., 231
Beyond Medicare, 239
Blood, Medicare coverage of, 40
Bloom, Jill, 228
Bone care, 157
Books, 227–236
BOSS (Benefits Outreach Screening Software), 258–259
Brand-name drugs, 144
Bridging the Medicare Gaps, 251–252
Brookdale Center on Aging, 162, 237
Budish, Armond D., 228
Buyer's Guide for supplemental insurance, 90
Buyer's Guide to Long Term Care, 258
Buyer's Guide to Medicare Supplemental Insurance for Californians, 241
Buying plans, 170

CACSC (California Association for Concerned Senior Citizens), 95
California Department of Insurance, 241
Can You Afford Nursing Home Care?, 245–246
Canada, Medicare coverage in, 22
Cancer Insurance Facts To Help You, 249
CAPS (Children of Aging Parents), 217
Carper, Jean, 228
Carriers, Medicare
   in appeals process, 76, 78
   list of, 178–183
   for Part B Medicare claims, 55
Case Management Resource Guide, 229
Case managers for home health services, 117, 215
Catastrophic insurance policies, 109
Catholic Charities U.S.A. (CCUSA), 214
Center for Consumer Healthcare Information, 229
Center for Medicare Advocacy, 223
Center for Public Representation (CPR), 162–163
Charges, Medicare, determination of, 59
Checklist for Comparing Long-Term Care Insurance, 237
Checklist for Purchasing Medicare Supplement Health Insurance, 237
Children of Aging Parents (CAPS), 217
Chiropractors, 38, 157
Choosing an HMO, 236
Chore home health services, 118–120
Chronic health problems, 31
Civil complaints for Part A Medicare appeals, 66
CLAIM (Community Leaders Assisting the Insured of Missouri), 224, 249
Clean sheeting by sales agents, 96
Clinical laboratory services, 39–40
Clinics, fraudulent, 145–146
CMP (Competitive Medical Plans), 97
Coinsurance
   for inpatient hospital services, 22, 23
   for Part B Medicare, 35, 44–45
   for skilled-nursing facilities, 28
   supplemental insurance for, 88, 93
   with VA benefits, 108
Collection of Medicare payments, 51–57
Commerce Clearing House, 240
Commissioner of Insurance (Nevada), 251
Commonwealth of Pennsylvania, 253–254
Community Leaders Assisting the Insured of Missouri (CLAIM), 224, 249
Comparison of Long-Term Care Insurers, 253–254
Competitive Medical Plans (CMP), 97
The Complete & Easy Guide to Social Security & Medicare, 231
The Complete Handbook of U.S. Government Benefits, 233
Comprehensive Outpatient Rehabilitation Facility Services (CORF), 39

Congressional committees, 193
Congressional Voting Record, 168
Conservatorships, 123–124
Consumer Guide, book by, 229
Consumer Long-Term Care Comparison Chart, 246
Consumer Protection, Connecticut Department of, 242
Consumer Protection Amendments (NAIC), 90–91
Consumer Reports articles, 239
The Consumer's Guide to Long-Term Care Insurance, 238
Consumer's Guide to Long-Term Care Insurance and Nursing Home Insurance in Maine, 246
A Consumer's Guide to Long Term Care Insurance in Vermont, 257
The Consumer's Guide to Medicare Supplemental Insurance, 238
Consumer's Guide to Social Security Benefits Including Medicare, 227–228
Copayments. *See* Coinsurance
CORF (Comprehensive Outpatient Rehabilitation Facility Services), 39
Cost contracts, 101
Cost of health care
    for home health coverage, 32, 113
    for hospice coverage, 34
    for hospitalization, 21
    for inpatient hospital services, 23
    in 1989, 6
    for nursing-home care, 27
    for Part B Medicare, 44–45
    for physician services, 36
    saving on, 139–146
    sharing of, 8, 44
    for skilled-nursing-facilities care, 28
Counseling programs, state, 221–225
Courts
    home health care coverage ruling by, 31
    for Part A Medicare appeals, 66
Coverage
    of home health care, 32
    of hospice care, 34
    of inpatient hospital services, 22–23
    with long-term insurance policies, 136
    by Medicaid, 106–107
    of physician services, 37–41
    of skilled-nursing facilities, 28
    of supplemental insurance, 90

CPR (Center for Public Representation), 162–163
Crichton, Jean, 229
Curran, Thomas, 97
Custodial care, 8, 28, 129
Customary charges, 59

Daily rule for skilled-nursing facilities, 27
Day care, 124, 213
Death and unpaid medical bills, 58, 60–61, 143
Death with dignity. *See* Hospice care and services
Deductibles
    and HMOs, 96
    for inpatient hospital services, 22, 23
    with long-term insurance policies, 136
    for Part B Medicare, 35, 43, 55
    supplemental insurance for, 88, 92
Deductions, tax, 141–143
Deluxe supplemental insurance policies, 92
Demand billing for Part A Medicare services, 65
    for home health care, 32, 75
    for SNF care, 29
Dental hygienists, 155
Dependent care, tax deductions for, 142–143
Developments in Aging, 193
Diagnostic categories, Medicare, 70–71
Diagnostic Related Group (DRG), 66, 70–73
Diagnostic X-ray services, 40
Dietitians, 158
Directory of Accredited/Approved Homemaker-Home Health Aide Services, 212
Directory of Diocesan Agencies of Catholic Charities in the U.S., Puerto Rico and Canada, 214
Directory of Member Agencies (FSA), 214
The Directory of Visiting Nurse Associations in the United States, 216
Disability and Medicare, 10, 16
Discharge from hospital, appealing of, 66, 70–73
Doctors. *See* Part B Medicare coverage; Physicians
Dread-disease policies, 109
DRG (Diagnostic Related Group), 66, 70–73
Drugs, saving on, 144–145
Duplication of supplemental insurance policies, 96
Durable medical equipment, 40

Early hospital discharges, 66, 70–73
Elder Affairs (Massachusetts), 247–248
Eldermed America (EMA), 163
Eligibility
    for Medicare, 9–10, 78, 82
    for Medicare HMOs, 101–103
Ellis, Junius, 232
Ellison, James W., 230
EMA (Eldermed America), 163
Emergency centers, ambulatory, 143–144
Emergency response systems (ERSs), 121
Enrollment
    in Medicare, 9–10, 45–48
    in Medicare HMOs, 102
EOMB (Explanation of Medicare Benefits),
    57, 59, 75–76
Equipment, Medicare coverage of, 40
ERSs (emergency response systems), 121
Escort home health services, 120–121
Evaluating Nursing Home Insurance,
    243–244
Excess charge billing, 49, 248
Exclusions with supplemental insurance, 93,
    137
Exercise programs, 127
Expenses, tax deductible, 141–142
Explanation of Medicare Benefits (EOMB),
    57, 59, 75–76
Eye care, 156, 215–216

Fabiola, 36
Families USA Foundation, 134–135,
    163–164
Family practitioners, 153
Family Service America (FSA), 214
Federal District Courts, 66
Federal Information Centers (FICs), 171–173
FHH (Foundation for Hospice and
    Homecare), 202, 212
*Filling in the Gaps: Health Insurance for
    People with Medicare,* 242
Filling the Medicare Gaps, 248–249
*Finances after 50: Financial Planning for the
    Rest of Your Life,* 234–235
Financial Planning for Long-Term Care, 234
Firman, James, 134
Fixed fee schedules, 45
Florida Department of Insurance, 243
Food stamps for home-delivered meals, 120
Foot care, 157
Forand, Aime, 6

Form HA-520 (Request for Review of
    Hearing Decision/Order), 66, 69
Form HA-5011 (Request for Hearing), 65, 68
Form HCFA-18 F5 (Application To Purchase
    Medicare Coverage), 11–15
Form HCFA-40B (Application for
    Enrollment in Medicare), 46–48
Form HCFA-1490S (Request for Medical
    Payment), 52–54
Form HCFA-1660 (Request for
    Information—Medicare Payment for
    Services to a Patient Now Deceased), 58,
    60–61
Form HCFA-1964 (Request for Review of
    Part B Medicare Claim), 76–77
Form HCFA-1965 (Request for
    Hearing—Part B Medicare Claim),
    78–79
Form HCFA-2649 (Request for
    Reconsideration of Part A Benefits), 65,
    67
Form SSA-1696 (Agreement To Have
    Representation at Hearing), 78, 80–81
Form SSA-3596 (Medicare Medical
    Insurance Claims Record), 55–56
Foster care, 123
Foundation for Hospice and Homecare
    (FHH), 202, 212
Fraud
    by clinics and physicians, 145–146
    by insurance salesmen, 90–91, 94–96
Free-look periods for supplemental
    insurance, 90, 137
Free-standing emergency centers, 143–144
Friendly visiting home health services, 120
FSA (Family Service America), 214

General Hospital, 20
Generic drugs, 144
Georgia Insurance Department, 243
Georgia Nursing Home Insurance Facts, 243
Geriatric clinics, 51
*Getting the Most from Social Security,
    Medicare and Other Government
    Benefits,* 229
GHAA (Group Health Association of
    America), 202
Government agencies, 171–193
Group buying plans, 170
Group Health Association of America
    (GHAA), 202

Group health insurance, 62
  evaluation of, 95
  as supplemental insurance, 87–88, 110
Guardianships, 123–124
Guide to Health Insurance for People with Medicare, 237
Guide to Long Term Care Insurance, 249
A Guide to Long-Term Care Insurance in the State of Oregon, 253
Guide to Nursing Home (Long-Term Care) Insurance, 251

A Handbook on the History and Issues of Health Care Services for the Elderly, 233
Handbooks, Medicare, 17–18, 173, 168, 238
Hanson, Stuart P., 227
HCFA (Health Care Financing Administration), 5, 16, 173, 237–238
Health Advocacy Services (HAS), 161
Health Benefits for an Aging Workforce, 170
Health Care and Finances: A Guide for Adult Children and Their Parents, 236–237
Health Care Education Associates, books by, 230
Health Care Financing Administration (HCFA), 5, 16, 173, 237–238
Health Care USA, 228–229
Health Insurance Advice for Senior Citizens, 258
Health Insurance Alternative, A Complete Guide to Health Maintenance Organizations, 232
Health Insurance and the Senior Citizen, 250
Health Insurance Association of America (HIAA), 164, 238
Health Insurance Continuation, 170, 238
Health Insurance Counseling and Advocacy Program (HICAP), 221
Health Insurance Facts To Help Senior Citizens, 249
Health Insurance Guide for Senior Citizens, 257
Health Letter, 239–240
Health Maintenance Organization Act, 97
Health maintenance organizations (HMOs), 86, 247
  books on, 228, 232
  listing of approved, 98–100
  Medicare claims submission by, 55
  organization for, 202

  pamphlets on, 236, 237
  for supplemental insurance, 96–103
Health Maintenance Organizations, 247
Health Promotion and Aging: A National Directory of Selected Programs, 169
Health-promotion techniques, 140–141, 169
Hearing care, 158–159
Hearings for Medicare claims, 65, 68, 76, 78–79
HIAA (Health Insurance Association of America), 164, 238
HICAP (Health Insurance Counseling and Advocacy Program), 221
High option long-term insurance policies, 135–136
History of Medicare, 6–8, 233
HMOs. *See* Health maintenance organizations
Home-equity conversions for long-term care, 138
Home health aides, 118, 159
Home health care and services
  appealing of claims for, 75
  associations for, 202–206, 212, 214–215
  directory for, 233
  HMOs for, 102
  insurance for, 136–137
  Medicare coverage of, 8, 29–33, 38
  noninstitutional services for, 116–117
  organization for, 202
  services for, 117–128
  sources of coverage for, 113–116
HomeCare News, 212
Homemaker–home health aides and services, 118–119, 159
Homer, 36
Homes, transferring of, 131
Hospice Benefits under Medicare, 237
Hospice care and services, 33–34
  appealing of claims for, 75
  directory for, 233
  as home health service, 121–122
  organizations for, 202, 212
  pamphlet on, 237
Hospital care
  appealing of discharges from, 66, 70–73
  indemnity policies for, 109
  inpatient, 20–26
  outpatient, 39
  VA, 108
  See also Part A Medicare coverage

Hospital Insurance Trust Fund, 6
House of Representatives Select Committee on Aging, 193
Housing, organizations for, 194–198
Housing and Urban Development, Department of, 133
Housing Options and Services for Older Adults: A Reference Handbook, 133, 138
How Do I Pay for My Long-Term Health Care?, 227
How To Keep Control of Your Life after 60, 232
How To Plan Your Successful Retirement, 227
How To Recover Your Medical Expenses, 236
How To Start a Self-Help Group for Caregivers, 217
Huber, Ezra, 234

IHPP (Intergovernmental Health Policy Project), 164, 240
Impersonation by sales agents, 96
An Important Message from Medicare, 23–25
In-home service workers, 118
Indemnity insurance policies, 109
Individual insurance policies, 110
Information and referral services, 116–117
Information Services (Texas), 255–256
Inlander, Charles B., 230
Inpatient hospital care, 20–26
Institute on Law and Aging, 126
Institute on Law and Rights of Older Adults, 162
Insurance. *See* Supplemental insurance
Insurance, Department of (New Jersey), 251
Insurance and Finance, Department of (Oregon), 253
Insurance commissions, 173–177
Insurance Dictionary, 235
Insurance Fraud Advice for Older Missourians, 250
Insurance Needs for Recipients of Medicare (INFORM): Consumer Guide, 230
Insurance Needs for Recipients of Medicare (INFORM): Workshop Guide, 230
Intergovernmental Health Policy Project (IHPP), 164, 240
Intermediaries, 32

Intermediate home health services, 118
Internal Revenue Service (IRS), 177–178
Internists, 153
Iowa Department of Elder Affairs, 244
Iowa Senior Citizens' Handbook, 244
I&R (information and referral) services, 116–117
IRS (Internal Revenue Service), 177–178
Is Medicare Enough?—A Shoppers' Guide to Supplemental Medical Insurance, 251
Itemized bills for Part B Medicare claims, 52

JCAHO (Joint Commission on Accreditation of Healthcare Organizations), 33, 207
Jehle, Faustin F., 231
Johnson, Lyndon Baines, 7
Joint Commission on Accreditation of Healthcare Organizations (JCAHO), 33, 207

Kaiser, Henry, 97
Kaiser-Permanente group plan, 97
Kansas Cancer Insurance Facts To Help You, 244
Kansas Health Insurance Facts To Help Senior Citizens, 244–245
Kansas Long Term Care Shopper's Guide, 245
Kansas Medicare Supplemental Insurance Shopper's Guide, 245
Kapp, Marshall B., 231
Kennedy, John F., 7
Kentucky Association of Health Care Facilities, 245
Kerr-Mills Act, 7
Kidney disease and Medicare, 10, 16
Kingson, Eric, 231
Knowing Your Rights, 236
Koski, Andrew, 237

Laboratory services, 39–40
LAMP (Legal Assistance to Medicare Patients), 223
LCE (Legal Counsel for the Elderly), 164–165, 238
Legal Aspects of Health Care for the Elderly: An Annotated Bibliography, 231
Legal Assistance to Medicare Patients (LAMP), 223
Legal Counsel for the Elderly (LCE), 164–165, 238

Legal guardianships, 123–124
Legal services and assistance, 125–126
  books on, 231–234
  organizations for, 164–166, 169, 223
Legal Services Corporation (LSC), 125–126,
  165–166
Legal Services of Middle Tennessee, Inc.,
  255
Liens on property and Medicaid, 132–133
Life insurance for long-term care, 138
Lifetime benefits with supplemental
  insurance, 93
Lifetime reserve for inpatient hospital
  services, 23
Limits on expenditures with supplemental
  insurance, 93
Lincoln National Corporation, 138
Long-Term Care: A Survival Guide,
  247–248
Long Term Care Campaign, 166
*Long Term Care Insurance: A Consumer
  Guide for Californians,* 241
Long-Term Care Insurance Buyer's Guide,
  250–251
Long-Term Care Standards Manual, 207
Long-term health care, 111
  assisted-living centers for, 133
  books for, 227, 234
  cost of, 8
  guides to, 241, 245–254, 256–258
  at home, 113–128
  insurance for, 133–138
  Medicare coverage for, 28
  need for, 112
  pamphlets for, 236–238
  retirement communities for, 133
  See also Nursing-home care and services
Loss ratios for supplemental insurance,
  91–92
Low option long-term insurance policies,
  135–136
LSC (Legal Services Corporation), 125–126,
  165–166

McClure, Grace, 121
McKay, Charles K., 230
McKernan, William John, 95
Madrzyk, Ana, 126
Mail carriers, reassurance services by, 121
Maine Committee on Aging, 246
Major medical insurance policies, 109

*Making the Most of Medicare: A Guide
  through the Medicare Maze,* 233–234
Managing Your Health Care Finances, 235
Marquardt, Dick, 257
Maryland Office on Aging, 247
Matthews, Joseph L., 231
Maximum benefits with supplemental
  insurance, 93
Mayer, Gloria Gilbert, 232
Mayer, Thomas R., 232
MCCA (Medicare Catastrophic Coverage
  Act), 7–8
Meals-on-wheels home health service, 120
Medicaid, 104–107
  enactment of, 7
  for home health care, 114
  and nursing home costs, 130
  offices for, 183–188
  and transfer of assets, 131–133
Medicaid buy in, 86, 107
Medical equipment and supplies, 40–41
Medical Insurance Assistance, Inc. (MIA),
  221–222
Medical specialists, 154
Medicare, 5
  appeals process for. *See* Appeals, Medicare
  assistance programs for, 16–17
  carriers for, 178–183
  costs and reimbursements of, 17, 43–45
  and death of beneficiary, 58, 60–61
  determination of charges in, 59
  and disability benefits, 10, 16
  eligibility for, 9–10
  handbook for, 17–18, 173, 238
  history of, 6–8, 233
  for home health care, 115
  limitations of, 8–9
  vs. Medicaid, 104
  notice of payments by, 57–58
  Part A. *See* Part A Medicare coverage
  Part B. *See* Part B Medicare coverage
  as secondary payer, 62
  supplementing of. *See* Supplemental
    insurance
Medicare and Employer Health Plans, 237
Medicare and Medicaid Guide, 240
Medicare & Medigap, 247
Medicare and Prepayment Plans, 237
Medicare Ban on Balance Billing Law, 248
Medicare Benefit Notice, 51, 57
Medicare Catastrophic Coverage Act, 7–8

Medicare Claims Information notice, 57–58
The Medicare Handbook, 17–18, 173, 238
Medicare Handbook (National Consumers
  League), 168, 238
Medicare Made Easy, 230
*Medicare, Medicaid, and Medicare
  Supplement Insurance: What You Need
  To Know To Protect Yourself,* 255
Medicare Medicaid Assistance Program
  (MMAP), 16–17, 161
*Medicare/Medicaid Nursing Home
  Information* guide, 129–130
Medicare Medical Insurance Claims Record,
  55–56
Medicare Misunderstandings, 248
Medicare—1989, 237
*Medicare-Participating Physicians/Supplier
  Directory,* 50
Medicare Series, 238
*Medicare Supplement Insurance: A Guide
  for Texas Consumers,* 255–256
*Medicare Supplemental Insurance
  Comparison Chart,* 246
*Medicare Supplemental Insurance in New
  York State,* 252
*Medicare Supplemental Insurance Shoppers'
  Guide,* 243
Medicare Training Manual, 242
Medigap Counseling Software, 259
Medigap Hotline (Wisconsin), 225
Medigap insurance. *See* Supplemental
  insurance
Medpard, 50
Menninger Clinic, 124
Mental-health services, 39, 157
Mexico, Medicare coverage in, 22
MIA (Medical Insurance Assistance, Inc.),
  221–222
Mieners, Mark, 133
Mills, Wilbur, 7
Minnesota Legal Services Coalition, 248
Mississippi Department of Insurance, 249
MMAP (Medicare Medicaid Assistance
  Program), 16–17, 161
Modern Maturity, 161
Money Magazine Editors, book by, 232
Money 1989, 232
*Montana Buyer's Guide to Medicare
  Supplemental Insurance,* 250
Montefiore Hospital, 29

Monthly premiums for Part B Medicare, 10,
  16, 43–46
Multipurpose senior centers, 124–125
Muscle care, 157
Myers, Teresa Schwab, 232

N4A (National Association of Area Agencies
  on Aging), 207
NAHC (National Association for Home
  Care), 31, 214–215, 233
NAIC (National Association of Insurance
  Commissioners), 90–91, 166–167, 173
NARP (National Association of Retired
  Persons), 95
NASUA (National Association of State Units
  on Aging), 207–211
NASW (National Association of Social
  Workers), 215
National Association for Home Care
  (NAHC), 31, 214–215, 233
National Association of Area Agencies on
  Aging (N4H), 207
National Association of Insurance
  Commissioners (NAIC), 90–91,
  166–167, 173
National Association of Private Geriatric
  Case Managers, 117, 215
National Association of Retired Persons
  (NARP), 95
National Association of Social Workers
  (NASW), 215
National Association of State Units on Aging
  (NASUA), 207–211
National Citizens Coalition for Nursing
  Home Reform (NCCNHR), 167
National Consumers League, 167–168, 238
National Council for Homemaker–Home
  Health Aide Services, 159, 202
National Council of Senior Citizens (NCSC),
  168
National Council on the Aging, Inc.
  (NCOA), 124, 168–169
National Eye Care Project (NECP), 215–216
National Federation of Licensed Practical
  Nurses (NFLPN), 216
National health insurance proposals, 6–8
National Health Law Program (NHLP), 169
National Home Care Directory, 215
National Homecaring Council (NHC), 119,
  202, 212

National Hospice Association (NHO), 212
National Institute of Senior Centers (NISC), 212
National Institute on Adult Daycare (NIAD), 124, 213
National Institute on Aging (NIA), 139–140
National League for Nursing (NLN), 216
National Library Project, 165
National Senior Citizens Law Center (NSCLC), 126, 169
National Support in Protective Services Law, 165
National Training Project, 165
NCCNHR (National Citizens Coalition for Nursing Home Reform), 167
NCOA (National Council on the Aging, Inc.), 124, 168–169
NCSC (National Council of Senior Citizens), 168
Nebraska Department of Insurance, 250
NECP (National Eye Care Project), 215–216
Neuman, R. Emil, 233
New information as basis of Medicare appeal, 78
NF (nursing facilities), 128–129
NFLPN (National Federation of Licensed Practical Nurses), 216
NHC (National Homecaring Council), 119, 202, 212
NHLP (National Health Law Program), 169
NHO (National Hospice Association), 212
NIA (National Institute on Aging), 139–140
NIAD (National Institute on Adult Daycare), 124, 213
1990 National Homecare and Hospice Directory, 233
NISC (National Institute of Senior Centers), 212
NLN (National League for Nursing), 216
No-payment billing for Part A Medicare services, 65
    for home health care, 32, 75
    for SNF care, 29
Noncoverage notices for hospital services, 72–74
Noninstitutional services for home health care, 116–117
North Central Regional Extension Publications, 243
North Dakota Insurance Department, 252

Not medically necessary noncoverage notices, 74
Notice of Noncoverage, 72–74
Notice of payments by Medicare, 57–58
Notice to Applicant Regarding Replacement Insurance, 90–91
NSCLC (National Senior Citizens Law Center), 126, 169
Nurses, 155, 216
Nursing care, 118
Nursing facilities (NF), 128–129
Nursing-home care and services, 128–133
    article on, 239
    book on, 228
    guides to, 243–246, 251–252
    and Medicare, 8
    need for, 112
    organization for reform of, 167
    and SNF, 26–27
    VA, 108
    See also Long-term health care
Nursing Home Insurance Shoppers Guide, 252
Nutrition home health services, 125

OAA. See Older Americans Act
Occupational therapists, 39, 158
Office of the Commissioner of Insurance (Wisconsin), 258
Ohio Buyer's Guide to Medicare Supplemental Health Insurance and Benefits Comparison Booklet, 253
Ohio Department of Insurance, 253
Older Americans Act (OAA)
    and day care, 124
    for home health care, 114
    for legal services, 126
    meals funded by, 120, 125
    and senior centers, 124–125
Older Women's League (OWL), 169, 238
Ombudsmen for long-term care, 127–128
Open-enrollment period
    for Medicare, 45
    for Medicare HMOs, 102
Ophthalmologists, 156
Opticians, 156
Optometrists, 38, 156
Organizations, directory of 161–225
    for counseling programs, 221–224
    general, 161–170

Organizations, directory of *(contintued)*
  government, 171–193
  health, social services, and long-term care, 194–213
  professional, 213–216
  self-help, 217–221
Orthopedists, 157
Out-of-pocket health-care costs, 87, 93
Outline of Coverage for supplemental insurance, 90
Outpatient hospital services, 39
OWL (Older Women's League), 169, 238

Pamphlets, 236–238
Paralegals, 126
Part A Medicare coverage, 17–20
  appealing of claims in, 64–75, 78–83
  collection of payments in, 51
  and death of beneficiary, 58, 60–61
  financing of, 6
  home health care, 29–33
  hospice care, 33–34
  inpatient hospital care, 20–26
  notice of payments by, 57–58
  skilled-nursing-facility care, 26–29
Part B Medicare coverage, 17–18, 35–41
  appealing of claims in, 64, 75–83
  assignment method with, 46, 49–51, 102, 145
  collection of payments in, 51–57
  costs of, 44–45
  and death of beneficiary, 58, 60–61
  enrolling in, 9–10, 45–48
  notice of payments by, 57–58
Participating physicians, 50–51
Payments, Medicare, collection of, 51–57
Pearman, William A., 233
Peer Review Organization (PRO), 22, 23
  and early hospital discharges, 72–73
  list of, 188–192
  pamphlet on, 236
  and preadmission notices of noncoverage, 74
  retrospective reviews by, 74
  and second surgical opinions, 38
  and SNF, 27
Pell, Arthur R., 233
Periodicals, 239–240
Personal home health services, 118
Physical fitness programs, 127

Physical therapists, 39, 158
Physician assistants, 154
Physicians, 36–41
  appealing of claims for services of, 75–78
  fraudulent, 145–146
  participating, 50–51
  types of, 153–154
  See also Part B Medicare coverage
Podiatrists, 38, 157
Policy replacement with supplemental insurance, 90–91, 94, 96
Portable diagnostic X-ray services, 40
PPOs (Preferred Provider Organizations), 103–104
PPS (prospective payment system), 66, 70–72, 236
A Practical Guide for Medigap Policies Offered in Utah, 256
Practices, insurance, 92–94
Preadmission notice of hospital noncoverage, 73–74
Preexisting conditions and supplemental insurance, 90–91, 93
Preferred Provider Organizations (PPOs), 103–104
Premiums
  Part B Medicare, 10, 16, 43–46
  for supplemental insurance, 89
Prescription drugs, saving on, 144–145
Prevailing charges, 59
Preventing Medigap Abuse, 241
Preventive health care and Medicare, 9
Private case managers for home health services, 117, 215
Private insurance. *See* Supplemental insurance
PRO. *See* Peer Review Organization
Professional organizations, 213–216
Prospective payment system (PPS), 66, 70–72, 236
Prosthetic devices, 40–41
Protective services, 123–124
Prudential Insurance Co. of America, 138
Psychiatrists, 157
Psychologists, 157
Public Citizen Health Research Group, 239

Qualifications
  for home health care, 30–31
  for hospice care, 33

Qualifications *(continued)*
  for inpatient hospital services, 21–22
  for skilled-nursing-facility coverage, 27
Quality Care Advocate, 167

Railroad Retirement and Medicare, 5, 9–10
Reasonable and necessary care, 9
Reconsiderations of Medicare claims, 65
Records of Part B Medicare expenses, 55–56
Regan, John J., 234
Registered dietitians, 158
Registered nurses, 155
Regulation of supplemental insurance,
  91–92
Renewability of supplemental insurance, 91,
  94, 137
Representative Payee Project, 165
Request for Hearing, 65, 68
Request for Hearing—Part B Medicare
  Claim, 78–79
Request for Information—Medicare
  Payment for Services to a Patient Now
  Deceased, 58, 60–61
Request for Medical Payment, 52–54
Request for Reconsideration for Part A
  Benefits, 65, 67
Request for Review of Hearing
  Decision/Order, 66, 69
Request for Review of Part B Medicare
  Claim, 77
Request for Social Security Appeals Council
  Review, 69
Reserve days for inpatient hospital services,
  23
Respite home health services, 122
Retired Senior Volunteer Program (RSVP),
  222
Retirement
  communities for, 133
  planning for, 227, 230
Retiring on Your Own Terms, 230
Retrospective reviews, 74
The Revolution in Health Care HMOs, 228
Rhode Island Department of Elderly Affairs,
  254
*Rhode Island Guide to Buying Medicare
  Supplemental Insurance,* 254
Rights of patients
  in hospital, 71–72
  in nursing homes, 130

Risk contracts, 97, 101
Risk factors for nursing homes, 128
Robert Wood Johnson Foundation, 133, 136
RSVP (Retired Senior Volunteer Program),
  222
Rubin, Leona G., 234

Saving on health costs, 139–146
Scare tactics by sales agents, 96
Schneider, Ira S., 234
Second surgical opinions, 37–38, 143
Secondary payer, Medicare as, 62
Select Committee on Aging, 193
Self-Help Center, 217
Self-Help Clearinghouse, 218–221
Self-Help Source Book, 218
Self-help support groups and organizations,
  126–127, 217–221
Senate Special Committee on Aging, 7, 193
Senior Center Report, 212
Senior centers, 124–125
Senior Citizens News, 168
Senior Health Insurance Benefits Advisors
  (SHIBA), 225
Senior Health Insurance Counseling Program
  (SHIC-P), 222, 242
Senior Health Insurance Programs (SHIP),
  223–224
Serving Health Information Needs of Elders
  (SHINE), 223–224
Shane, Dorlene V., 234
SHIBA (Senior Health Insurance Benefits
  Advisors), 225
SHIC-P (Senior Health Insurance Counseling
  Program), 222, 242
SHINE (Serving Health Information Needs
  of Elders), 223–224
SHIP (Senior Health Insurance Programs),
  223–224
*A Shopper's Guide to Long Term Care
  Insurance in Texas,* 256
Skilled nursing care, 118
Skilled-nursing-facility (SNF) care, 26–29, 75
Social Security
  books on, 227–229, 231–232, 234
  and Medicare, 5, 9–10, 16, 44, 173
Social Security Administrative Hearing, 65,
  68
Social Security Appeals Council Review, 66,
  69

Social Security, Medicare and Pensions, 231–232

Social Service Block Grants (SSBG), 115

Social Work Directory, 215

Social workers, 159, 215

Software, 258–259

South Carolina Department of Insurance, 255

South Carolina Health Insurance Buyer's Guide, 255

Special-enrollment period for Part B Medicare, 45–46

Special Investigative Unit, 250

Specified-disease policies, 109

Speech-language services, 39, 158–159

Spells of illness for inpatient hospital services, 23

Spitzer-Resnick, Jeffrey, 235

Sporkin, Stanley, 31

Spousal impoverishment protection, 132

SSBG (Social Service Block Grants), 115

Standard supplemental insurance policies, 92

Standards
  for Medicare services, 9
  for supplemental insurance, 89–91

Starr, P., 233

State Health Notes, 240

State insurance commissions, regulation by, 91–92

State of Montana Insurance Commission, 250

State of New Hampshire Insurance Department, 251

State of New York Insurance Department, 252

State Units on Aging (SUA), 114–115, 207–211

States
  AAHA associations in, 194–198
  AHCA associations in, 198–201
  counseling programs in, 221–224
  Federal Information Centers in, 171–173
  home health care associations in, 202–206
  insurance commissions in, 173–177
  Medicaid offices in, 183–188
  Medicare carriers in, 178–183
  PROs in, 188–192
  publications by, 241–258
  self-help clearinghouses in, 218–221
  SUAs in, 207–211

SUA (State Units on Aging), 114–115, 207–211

Supplementing Medicare, 85–86
  catastrophic insurance, 109
  group health insurance, 87–88
  guides to, 241–243, 245–258
  HMOs, 96–103
  for home health care, 116
  indemnity, 109
  for long-term care, 133–138
  for low-income beneficiaries, 107
  Medicaid for, 104–107
  pamphlets on, 237–238
  policy replacement, 90–91, 94, 96
  PPOs, 103–104
  purchasing insurance, 88–96
  submission of claims for, 52, 57–58
  veterans' benefits as, 107–108

Supplementing Medicare, 248

Supplies, Medicare coverage of, 41

Support groups, 126–127

Surgical opinions, Medicare coverage of, 37–38, 143

Switching of policies by sales agents, 96

Tax Counseling for the Elderly program, 177–178

Tax credits and deductions, 141–143

Telephone reassurance home health services, 121

Tele-Tax service, 177

Terminal illnesses. *See* Hospice care and services

Theft by sales agents, 96

Therapists, 158

Thomsett, Michael, 235

Thrifty supplemental insurance policies, 92

Time limits for Medicare claims submissions, 55

Together on Aging, 170

Transfer of assets for Medicaid, 131–132

Transportation home health services, 122–123

Travel
  and HMO coverage, 103
  and Medicare coverage, 22–23

Trust funds, 6

Types
  of long-term insurance policies, 135–136
  of nursing homes, 128–130
  of supplemental insurance, 92

United Seniors Health Cooperative (USHC), 170, 235, 240, 259
United Seniors Health Report, 240
Urban Mass Transit Act, 122–123
URC. *See* Utilization Review Committee
U.S. Congress committees on aging, 193
USHC (United Seniors Health Cooperative), 170, 235, 240, 259
Utah Department of Insurance, 256
Utilization Review Committee (URC), 22, 23
   and early hospital discharges, 72
   and preadmission notices of hospital noncoverage, 73–74
   and SNF, 27

Vermont Office on Aging, 257
Veterans Affairs, Department of, 171
   and adult foster care, 123
   benefits from, 107–108
   and home health care, 116
Veterans of Foreign Wars, 108
Villers Foundation (Families USA Foundation), 163–164
Visiting home health services, 120
Visiting Nurse Association, 29
Visiting Nurse Associations of America (VNAA), 216

Waiting periods with supplemental insurance, 93, 137

Waiver of liability
   appealing denial of, 82–83
   and retrospective PRO reviews, 74
   for skilled-nursing facilities, 29
Walk-in emergency centers, 143–144
Waller, Kal, 236
Washington Business Group on Health (WBGH), 170
Welfare offices, 183–188
West Virginia Insurance Commissioner, 257
West Virginia Supplement Shopper's Guide, 257
Western Clinic, 97
What Insurance Policies Do Most Senior Citizens Need?, 252–253
What You Must Know about Social Security and Medicare, 231
Who Can Afford a Nursing Home?, 239
Wiener, Joshua, 134
Women, organizations for, 169–170, 238

X-ray services, 40

Yocum, James, 97
Your Guide to Long-Term Care Insurance, 254
Your Legal Rights in Later Life, 234
Your 1989/90 Guide to Social Security Benefits, 234
Your Real Medicare Handbook, 163, 235